'Harrowing, ▮▮▮▮▮▮▮▮'

KT-495-955

'An eye-opener'

'Christie Watson is a wonderful writer'

'Passionate, political, heart-breaking'

'Stunning'

'So honest, so wise... she writes beautifully'

'Compelling and universally relevant... A joy to read'

'Moving, eloquent, funny, inspiring'

'Touching, thought-provoking' *DAILY EXPRESS*

'Compelling'
NEW YORK TIMES

'Beautiful – tender, informative, unflinching'
RACHEL JOYCE

'Lyrical, moving'
STYLIST

'A message of self-compassion as useful for those of us outside the medical world, as in it'
JULIA SAMUEL

'Life-changing... A much needed human voice'
IRISH TIMES

'Elegant, fascinating, unforgettable'
SUNDAY EXPRESS

'An important book that should be on everyone's reading list' WOMAN & HOME

'Completely absorbing... uplifting, compassionate' THE TABLET

'Terrifically moving' SUNDAY TIMES

'Teeming with humanity' SUNDAY BUSINESS POST

'Astonishing' RED MAGAZINE

'Beautifully written' DAILY TELEGRAPH

'Amusing, hilarious, enthralling' THE ARTS DESK

'Poignant, powerful... A must-read for all nurses' PROFESSOR JANE CUMMINGS, CHIEF NURSING OFFICER ENGLAND

ALSO BY CHRISTIE WATSON

Tiny Sunbirds Far Away
Where Women are Kings

CHRISTIE WATSON

The Language of Kindness

A Nurse's Story

VINTAGE

5 7 9 10 8 6 4

Vintage
20 Vauxhall Bridge Road,
London SW1V 2SA

Vintage is part of the Penguin Random House group of companies
whose addresses can be found at global.penguinrandomhouse.com.

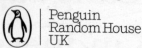
Penguin
Random House
UK

First published in the UK by Chatto & Windus in 2018
First published by Vintage in 2019

penguin.co.uk/vintage

A CIP catalogue record for this book is available from
the British Library

ISBN 9781784706883

Printed and bound in Great Britain by Clays Ltd, Elcograf S.p.A.

Penguin Random House is committed to a sustainable future
for our business, our readers and our planet. This book is
made from Forest Stewardship Council® certified paper.

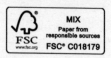
MIX
Paper from
responsible sources
FSC® C018179

For Nurses

A poet is a nightingale who sits in darkness, and sings to cheer its own solitude with sweet sounds; his auditors are as men entranced by the melody of an unseen musician, who feel that they are moved and softened, yet know not whence or why.

Percy Bysshe Shelley

Contents

Author's Note

The events described here are based on memories of my experiences as a nurse. The identifying features of people and places have been changed in order to protect the privacy of patients and colleagues and descriptions of certain individuals and situations have been merged to further protect identities. Any similarities are purely coincidental.

Introduction:
Worth Risking Life For

Nursing was left to 'those who were too old, too weak, too drunken, too dirty, too stupid or too bad to do anything else'.

Florence Nightingale

I didn't always want to be a nurse. I went through a number of career possibilities and continually exasperated the careers advisor at my failing secondary school. 'Marine biologist' was one career choice that I listed, having visions of wearing a swimsuit all day in a sunny climate and swimming with dolphins. When I discovered that much of the work of a marine biologist involved studying plankton off the coast of Wales, I had a rethink. During one summer in Swansea I spent time watching my great-great-aunt gutting catfish in the large kitchen sink; and once I went out on a boat with hairy, gruff and burly yellow-booted men who pissed in the sea and swore continually. I'd also eaten cockles and laver bread for breakfast. Marine biology was definitely out.

'Law,' a teacher remarked, when my parents, also exasperated with me by then, asked what I might be suited to. 'She can argue all day long.' But I had no aptitude for focused study.

Instead I looked towards other animals and conservation. I dreamed of doing photography for the *National Geographic*, leading to travel in hot and exotic locations where the sun would shine and I would wear a swimsuit all day after all, and live in flip-flops. I joined marches and anti-vivisection campaigns, and gave out leaflets in the grey-brick town centre of Stevenage showing pictures of dogs being tortured, rabbits having cosmetics tested on them until their eyes became red, and bloody, skeletal cats. I wore political badges that were outdoor-market cheap and came loose, stabbing me until one evening I found a tiny constellation of pin-prick bruises on my chest. I refused to go into the living room after my mum bought a stuffed chick from a car-boot sale and placed it amongst her ornaments, and instead ate my vegetarian dinner on the stairs in protest, saying, 'It's me or the chick. I cannot be associated with murder.'

My mum, with endless patience, constantly forgave my teenage angst, removed the chick, made me another cheese sandwich and gave me a hug. It was she who taught me the language of kindness, though I didn't appreciate it back then. The next day I stole a rat from school, to save it from dissection by the biology department. I called it Furter, and hoped it would live safely with my existing pet rat, Frank, which used to sit on my shoulder, its long tail swinging around me like a statement necklace. Of course, Frank ate Furter.

Swimmer, jazz trumpeter, travel agent, singer, scientist... Astronomy was a possibility until, at the age of twelve, I discovered that my dad, who had taught me the name of every constellation, had made it all up. I didn't tell him, though; I still let him point upwards and tell me his stories, with his enthusiasm for narrative bursting into the sky. 'There – the shape of a hippo? You see it? That's called Oriel's Shoulder. And that is the Bluebell. You see the shape? The almost silver-blue colour of those particular stars? Fishermen believe that if you look to the stars hard enough, they will whisper the secrets of the earth. Like hearing the secrets of the sea inside a shell. If you listen hard, you can hear nothing and everything, all at the same time.'

I spent hours and hours looking at the stars to hear the secrets of the earth. At night I pulled out a cardboard box full of treasures from underneath my bed: old letters, a broken key ring, my dead grandfather's watch, a single drachma; chewing gum that I had retrieved from underneath a desk, and which had been in the mouth of a boy I liked; stones I had collected from various places, and a large shell. I would stand in my bedroom looking up towards the stars, holding the shell to my ear.

One night, burglars came to steal meat from our freezer, which we kept in the garden shed. Those were the days when people bought meat in bulk at car-boot sales, from men on giant lorries with loudspeakers and dirty white aprons. Those were the days when police would come at night to investigate frozen-chicken theft, and my star-watching was interrupted by police shouting. The universe had answered my shell-call: vegetarianism mattered. I am not sure which would have been a more unusual sight that night: a few young men carrying a frozen chicken and a giant packet of lamb chops, or a skinny teenager in a moonlit bedroom, with a large shell pressed against her ear.

What I would do – and who I would be – consumed me in a way that didn't seem to worry my friends. I didn't understand then that I wanted to live many lives, to experience different ways of living. I didn't know then that I would find exactly what I searched for (minus the swimsuit and the sun): that both nursing and writing are about stepping into other shoes all the time.

From the age of twelve I always had part-time jobs. I worked in a café cleaning the ovens – a disgusting job, with mean women who used to make the teabags last three cups. I did a milk round, carrying milk during the freezing winter, until I could no longer feel my fingers. I did a paper round, until I was found dumping papers in dog-shit alley. I didn't make any effort at school; I did no homework. My parents tried to expand my horizons, give me ideas about what I might do and a work ethic: 'Education is a ticket to anywhere. You have a brilliant brain, but you don't want to use it.' I was naturally bright but, despite the tools my parents gave me and their *joie de vivre*, my poor school-work ethic and my flightiness continued. They always encouraged me to read, and I was consumed by philosophy, looking for answers to my many questions: Sartre, Plato, Aristotle, Camus – I was hooked. A love of books was the best gift they ever gave me. I liked to roam and not be far from reading material; I hid books around the estate: *Little Women* in the Black Alley; Dostoevsky behind Catweazel's bins; Dickens under Tinker's broken-down car.

I left school at sixteen and moved in with my twenty-something boyfriend and his four twenty-something male lodgers. It was unbelievably chaotic, but I was blissfully content working a stint at a video shop, handing out VHS videos to the Chinese takeaway next door in exchange for chicken chow mein, my vegetarianism now beginning to wane, as I concentrated on putting on 18-rated films in the shop and filling the place with my friends. I went to agricultural college to become a farmer and lasted two weeks. A BTEC in travel and tourism lasted a week. To say that I had no direction was an understatement.

I was truly devastated when, after turning up late for an interview, I did not get the job of children's entertainer at Pizza Hut. It was a shock when my relationship broke down, despite being only sixteen and completely naive. My pride meant that I would never go home. No job, no home. So

I worked for Community Service Volunteers, which was the only agency I could find at the time that accepted sixteen-year-olds instead of eighteen-year-olds and provided accommodation. I was sent to a residential centre run by the Spastics Society (now called Scope), earning £20 pocket money a week by looking after adults with severe physical disabilities: helping them to toilet, eat and dress. It was the first time I felt as if I was doing something worthwhile. I had begun eating meat and I had a bigger cause. I shaved my head and lived in charity-shop clothes, spending all my pocket money on cider and tobacco. I had nothing, but I was happy. And it was the first time I'd been around nurses. I watched the qualified nurses with the kind of intensity that a child watches her parents when she's sick. My eyes didn't leave them. I had no language for what they were doing, or for their job.

'You should do nursing,' one of them said. 'They give you a bursary and somewhere to live.'

I went to the local library and discovered an entire building full of waifs and strays like me. I had been to my school library, and to the library in Stevenage, many times when I was much younger, but this library was about more than simply learning and borrowing books. It was a place of sanctuary. There was a homeless man asleep, and the librarians left him alone. A woman on a mobility scooter was being helped by a man who had a sign round his neck that said he had autism and was there to help, reaching a book on a top shelf for her. There were children running around freely, and groups of younger teenagers huddled together, laughing.

I found out about Mary Seacole, who – like Florence Nightingale – nursed soldiers during the Crimean War. She began experimenting in nursing by administering medicine to a doll, and then progressed to pets, before helping humans. I hadn't considered nursing as a profession before, but then I began remembering: my brother and I purposefully ripped the stuffing out of soft toys or pulled the glass eyes from dolls, so that I could fix them. I remembered my primary-school classmates queuing for an anaemia check-up; I must have bragged about my specialist knowledge, before lining them up outside school and pulling down their eyelids, one by one, to see if they needed to eat liver and onions; and the endless friends with sore throats whose necks I would gently press with my fingertips, as if on a clarinet. 'Lymph node.'

There wasn't much written about what nursing involved, or how to go about it, so I had no idea whether or not I'd be suitable. I discovered that nursing pre-dates the history books and has long existed in every culture. One of the earliest written texts relating to nursing is the *Charaka-saṃhita*, which was compiled in India around the first century BC and stated that nurses should be sympathetic towards everyone. And nursing has strong links with Islam. In the early seventh

century, faithful Muslims became nurses – the first professional nurse in the history of Islam, Rufaidah bint Sa'ad, was
described as an ideal nurse, due to her compassion and
empathy.

Sympathy, compassion, empathy: this is what history tells
us makes a good nurse. I have often revisited in my head that
trip to the library in Buckinghamshire, as those qualities seem
to have been lacking all too often during my career – qualities
that we've now forgotten or no longer value. But, at sixteen,
I was full of hopeful energy and idealism. And when I turned
seventeen I decided to go for it. No more career choice changes
and flitting around; I would become a nurse. Plus, I knew
there would be parties.

A few months later, I somehow slipped onto a nursing
course, despite being younger by a couple of weeks than the
official entry age of seventeen-and-a-half. I moved into
nursing halls in Bedford. The halls were at the back of the
hospital, a large block of flats filled with the sound of banging
doors and occasional screaming laughter. Most of my corridor
was made up of first-year nurses, with a few radiographers
and physiotherapy students, plus the occasional doctor on
rotation. The student nurses were almost all young and wild,
and away from home for the first time. There were a significant number of Irish women ('we had two choices,' they'd
tell me, 'nurse or nun'); and a small number of men (universally gay at the time). There was a laundry room downstairs,

next to a stuffy television room with plastic-coated armchairs which the back of my legs stuck to, in the heat from the radiators on full blast twenty-four hours a day. I met a trainee psychiatrist in that television room, after inadvertently blurting out that I was stuck to the chair, and he became my boyfriend for a few years. My bedroom was next to the toilets and smelled of damp, and one of my friends once grew cress on the carpet. The kitchen was dirty and the fridge was full of out-of-date food, with a note on one cupboard stating: DO NOT STEAL OTHER PEOPLE'S FOOD. WE KNOW WHO YOU ARE.

There was one telephone in an echoing hallway, which rang at all hours of the day and night. There were arguments, and the sound of heels running and of music being played loudly. We all smoked – cigarettes usually, but the smell of weed was like a constant low-level background noise that you didn't even notice after a while. We went in and out of each other's rooms in a communal fashion, and our doors were never locked. In my room Leonardo da Vinci's anatomical drawings of the chambers of the heart were on a poster above my bed; there was a shelf full of nursing textbooks and tatty novels, and a pile of philosophy books next to my bed. Plus a kettle, a radiator that wouldn't turn down and a window that didn't open. There was a sink to wash in (bodies and cups), to flick ash in, to vomit in and, for a few weeks when the toilets were continuously blocked, to pee in. To my contemporaries, it wasn't much; but after sharing a room in the residential centre for so long, and previously a house with a boyfriend and his male lodgers, it was heaven to me.

The first night, though, is always the worst. I had no idea what I would be doing as a nurse, and had begun to regret not asking more questions of the nurses who had encouraged me to apply. I was terrified of failure; of the look on my parents' faces when I announced yet another change of heart. They had been shocked enough about my decision to become a nurse: my dad actually laughed out loud. Despite my work as a carer, they still saw me as the rebellious teenager who couldn't care less about anyone. It was a far stretch to imagine me being devoted to kindness.

I lay awake that night and listened to the sound of my immediate neighbour arguing with her boyfriend, a moody, lanky security guard who, against all the rules, appeared to be living with her. Even after they were quiet I couldn't sleep. My head was dancing with doubt. I knew I'd be class-room-based for a while at least, so I wouldn't kill anyone by accident, or have to wash an old man's penis or experience similar horrors. But I was full of anxiety. And when I went that night to the toilet, which was shared by those on the entire floor, I found a used sanitary towel stuck on the bathroom door. I retched. Aside from how vile it was, I remembered then that the sight of blood had always made me feel faint.

My queasy nature was confirmed the following morning when we had our occupational health screening. Blood samples were taken from all of us. 'To hold on file,' the phlebotomist announced. 'In case you get a needle-stick injury and contract HIV. We can then find out if you were HIV-positive already.' It was 1994, and misinformation and fear about HIV were everywhere. The phlebotomist tied a tourniquet around my arm. 'Are you a student nurse or a medical student?' she asked.

I watched the needle, the blood filling the tube, and the room began to blur. Her voice sounded far away.

'Christie. Christie!' When I came round, I was lying on the floor with my legs up on the chair, and the phlebotomist above me. She laughed. 'You okay now?'

I slowly got to my elbows, regaining focus. 'What happened?'

'You fainted, dear. Happens. Though you might want to rethink your career.'

Twenty years in nursing has taken so much from me, but has given me back even more. I want to share with you the tragedies and joys of a remarkable career. Come with me on the wards, from birth to death; past the Special-Care Baby Unit and the double doors to the medical ward; run through the corridors to answer the crash bleep, past the pharmacy and staff kitchen, and to Accident and Emergency. We will explore the hospital itself, as well as nursing in many of its aspects. What I thought nursing involved when I started: chemistry, biology, physics, pharmacology and anatomy. And what I now know to be the truth of nursing: philosophy, psychology, art, ethics and politics. We will meet people on the way: patients, relatives and staff – people you may recognise already. Because we are all nursed at some point in our lives. We are all nurses.

1

A Tree of Veins

Everyone has the right to a standard of living adequate for the health and well-being of himself and of his family, including food, clothing, housing and medical care.

Article 25 of the Universal Declaration of Human Rights

I walk across the bridge towards its jagged-edged shadow, watch the pale-blue, almost green, grey light dancing on the water below: it is dawn. Everything is quiet. A full moon. A couple of women swerve past me, wearing party clothes and smudged mascara; a man in a sleeping bag is slumped against the wall, a coffee cup beside his head containing a few coins. There is hardly any traffic, but for a few black cabs and the occasional night bus. But there are other people like me heading to the hospital: a uniform of scuffed flat shoes, rucksack, pale face, bad posture.

I turn into the hospital grounds and walk past the small church in the courtyard, which is always open. Inside, it is dark and lit by dull lighting and candles, with a book full of messages and prayer requests on the altar. The saddest book you will ever read.

The staff are rushing in through the main entrance; some pushing bikes, others walking with purpose, trying not to catch the eye of anyone anxiously searching for information, carrying a letter and an overnight bag, holding the hand of a crying child or pushing an elderly relative in a wheelchair, a blanket tucked over their knees. At 9 a.m. there will be a volunteer to help the lost, wearing a banner that reads: 'How Can I Help You?' This is Ken, who is seventy and whose granddaughter was treated at the hospital for sepsis, following treatment for ovarian cancer; 'I want to help people like me. It's the little things.' He gives out maps of the hospital layout, directions and a smile. The map of the hospital is colour-coded, and there are coloured stripes on the floor for people to follow. At least once a day someone will sing and skip as they follow the yellow stripe: 'We're off to see the wizard...'

I walk past the reception seating area, where even more people are huddled together: rich and poor, disabled and able-bodied, people of all races and cultures and ages. Often I see the same woman – wearing slippers and reeking of urine, sitting next to a trolley filled with plastic bags – muttering to herself. Sometimes she shouts out as if she's in pain, and a security guard's face will pop up at the hatch to check for disturbances, before disappearing again. But today she's not there. Instead I see an elderly woman wearing a thick red coat, despite the hospital heating. She looks up at me for a few seconds with frightened, sad eyes. She seems completely lost and alone despite the dozen or so people around her. Her hair, once curled, is now unwashed and half-flat; it reminds me of my nan's hair when she got sick, and how she hated not having a perfect blow-dry. She closes her eyes and rests her forehead on her hands.

I love walking through the hospital. Hospitals have always been places of sanctuary. King Pandukabhaya of Sri Lanka (who lived from 437 to 367 BC) built lying-in homes in various parts of his kingdom – the earliest evidence anywhere in the world of institutions dedicated specifically to the care of the sick. A psychiatric hospital was built in Baghdad in 805 AD. These early hospitals were forbidden by law to turn away patients who were unable to pay for care. The Qalawun Hospital in thirteenth-century Egypt stated: 'All costs are to be borne by the hospital, whether the people come from afar or near, whether they are residents or foreigners, strong or weak, low or high, rich or poor, employed or unemployed, blind or sighted, physically or mentally ill, learned or illiterate.'

I walk on, past the gift shop where 'Congratulations' and 'With Sympathy' cards are separated by 'Get Well Soon'. I pass the tiny clothes shop where nobody ever buys clothes, but the shopkeeper tells good stories and knows everything that is happening in the hospital; on to the public toilets where patients collapse, inject heroin and, occasionally, are attacked – once even raped. Opposite the toilets are the newsagent's and the twenty-four-hour café, where sour milk from the broken coffee machine once flooded onto the lifesaving defibrillators stored in the basement below.

I turn the corner and glance back at the woman in the thick red coat, nearly colliding with a kitchen assistant pushing a giant metal trolley which smells of bleach, mould and aeroplane food. Left of the coffee shop are the lifts where there is always a cluster of people waiting. The hospital is built on expensive land and grows vertically; most of the wards are above the main veins and arteries of the ever-expanding hospital buildings. But the long wards with their many windows are still recognisable as having the same architectural layout that Florence Nightingale suggested, recognising the role of good architecture and hospital design in improving patients' health. She recommended that ward layouts comprised of long, narrow blocks with tall windows, maximising the fresh air and sunlight. In her correspondence between 1865 and 1868 with the Manchester architect Thomas Worthington, Nightingale also highlighted the practical needs of the nurses: 'Will the Scullery be sufficient accommodation for a nurse to sleep in, if necessary?'

I imagine her footsteps, and watch my own as I pass the patient transport area, where there is an entire room full of people waiting to go home, too sick to travel by public transport and too poor to go by taxi; none of them have relatives to collect them. The patients are sitting in wheelchairs and plastic chairs, wearing coats or dressing gowns and blankets, looking at the automatic doors for the face of a stranger; looking past the automatic doors at the sky outside, its emptiness. The vending machine whirrs, untouched, behind the row of chairs. I wonder if these people – most of them elderly and frail – are hungry, or in pain, or frightened. I already know the answer. The waiting room to leave the hospital seems fuller than the waiting room to get in. Everything is relative. Patients may not feel lucky to suffer a serious injury and be fighting for their life in Accident and Emergency (A&E), but if they have family and friends with them, then maybe they are lucky.

The porters' lodge door opens and slams continually into a line of empty oxygen cylinders, looking like giant skittles. A woman with frizzy hair and drawn-on eyebrows has a Madonna-esque earpiece and microphone and a switchboard pad in front of her. She is someone I spend time trying to befriend. But despite my efforts she barks, 'Can I help you?' every time I say hello, as if I am a stranger. Still, I persist.

The pharmacy is next door: a giant sweet shop for adults. There are trays that pull out, and miles of lines of different tablets. The inside of the pharmacy is like a trading floor on Wall Street, down a low-lit staircase to the basement, where certain drugs are organised into emergency boxes, labelled whenever they are opened, to ensure they're not tampered with, then restocked and sealed. Many of the drugs are used in the UK without NICE (the National Institute for Health and Care Excellence) approval. This is not uncommon. In paediatric use in America, for example, only 20 to 30 per cent of drugs are FDA-approved.

Drug reps are salespeople, and they used to be a source of excitement in hospital. They are easy to spot; like the pharmacists, they are better dressed than the doctors. A uniform of designer clothing and the manner of a car salesman, plus the ability to get the attention of a busy consultant (and past the consultants' secretaries), mean that a good-looking undercover army of twenty- and thirty-year-old graduates, who didn't quite get the grades for medical school, regularly visit hospitals. A visit on the wards from the drug rep used to mean pizzas, pens, notebooks and other gifts. 'Transparency' means that the drug-rep lunches are now less luxurious, and doctors are not allowed to be bribed to stock or prescribe one particular drug over another. The reps still give out promotional material, though (all doctors and nurses have mugs and pens in their houses with the name of drugs on them, and for a long time my baby daughter had a favourite teddy bear that wore a T-shirt advertising an antidepressant).

There is a small hatch and a constant stream of student nurses waiting for TTO (To Take Out – a drug prescription that a patient is taking home, like a takeaway from a restaurant); and a door where you have to get buzzed in, for certain drugs or fluids.

My office is three floors above the pharmacy. It is an over-hot, over-stuffed, carpeted room with exposed pipes and rat-traps outside the door, but we're not in here much. I look around the room for a few seconds, my eyes sweeping the table, on which rest out-of-date endotracheal tubes and faulty defibrillator pads ('They were sparking, but it's anecdotal, so we don't need to panic yet!'). There are sachets of stolen brown sauce from the hospital canteen, where we stop occasionally for toast or fried breakfast, after receiving a handover from the site nurse practitioners (SNPs) – the senior nurses who manage the hospital overnight and deal with all manner of hospital issues, from bed management to critical incidents, security and terrorist attacks. Also on the table are the thick medical notes of a patient who died, waiting to go back to the bereavement office; plus a large tub of decaffeinated coffee, which I was told on my first day had been there, unused, for years.

My job as a resuscitation officer is a strange hybrid role – a specialist nurse expert at resuscitation. Our team is mostly staffed by experienced former intensive-care nurses (like me) or Accident and Emergency nurses, but sometimes by paramedics or operating department practitioners (highly trained operating-theatre assistants). We teach nurses and doctors and other healthcare professionals about resuscitation, and carry crash bleeps (or pagers) that take us to all areas of the hospital: the wards, theatres, coffee shop, stairwell, psychiatry outpatients, the car park and wards for the elderly; and we work with a team and help the staff manage medical emergencies and cardiac arrests.

I change behind a makeshift screen. There is no other place to change in our office, and no time to go to the toilets; the makeshift screens have been a feature for years. The crash bleep goes off, flashing and emitting an alarm: 'Adult Crash Call, Main Canteen'. The crash bleep can be silent all day. On other days it can go off five or six times. Staff put out the call by ringing 2222 and specifying the type of emergency: adult, paediatric, obstetric, neonatal or trauma. Even in hospital, medical emergencies can be rare, but may be also horrific, although most of the calls are what we quietly consider a load of nonsense: a patient who has fainted or is faking a seizure or, once, had been stung by a wasp.

'My advice,' a colleague tells me on my first day, 'is to run very, very slowly. You do not know what you will find, and you certainly don't want to be first on the scene until you know what you're doing.'

But now I've been doing the job for a while, so I respond into the bleep, 'Resus Officer', and run down the stairs two at a time, past the central area of the hospital, which is dominated by a giant statue of Queen Victoria. I run past the grand hallway, with the piano that is played by people who will surprise you. Today there is a builder in a high-visibility jacket playing Mozart. Past a slow-walking woman and a beaming man, pushing a dot of a baby in an immaculately new push-chair, balloons attached: 'Congratulations: a Boy!' I have to slow down as the people get thicker near the post room, where the sounds of swearing and a radio burst through the cubby-hole and an occasional arm flings mail to the queue waiting outside. I walk quickly towards the cash machine that never works, and the hospital canteen where staff with hangovers are eating their fried breakfast.

The woman with the sad eyes wearing the red coat is tiny and frail-looking. She is even smaller when the coat comes off. She's wearing a floral shirt underneath that has the buttons done up wrong. Her skin is crinkled and dry, her hair white and patchy. Her eyes are rheumy and her lips cracked; her half-flat hair smells sour. A wedding ring hangs on a silver necklace just above her collarbone. Her eyes flick from person to person and she is shaking. She is in the canteen, conscious and sitting on a chair, already surrounded by some of the crash team: a senior doctor, a junior doctor, an anaesthetist and an SNP. They do not look worried. The SNP, Tife, is a friend. She was an A&E nurse for many years. It is always reassuring to see her: she is as calm as ever. She has somehow found a blanket, which you would imagine is easy but never is, and is kneeling in front of the patient attaching a small sensor to her finger to record her oxygen levels.

'Morning!' Tife says.

'Hi. Sorry – I was just getting changed.'

The crash trolley arrives with a porter. It is called for as soon as a crash bleep goes off, and generally arrives at the same time as the team. On it rests an enormous amount of kit – an entire ward on wheels. There's oxygen, suction, a defibrillator, emergency drugs, and large bags containing everything under the sun from glucose monitoring kits to breathing equipment.

'Betty here has a bit of chest pain. All the obs are fine. She's very cold. Can you get a Tempa-Dot?' She turns to the doctors. 'We'll get her to A&E, if you need to go.'

'She needs a twelve-lead ECG,' the doctor says, and leaves before she notices the junior doctor rolling his eyes and muttering, 'You think?' under his breath.

'Can I hand over to you?' he asks me as he runs. They have busy jobs as well as being on the crash team, and have to drop everything when the bleep goes off, sometimes leaving patients in theatre with only junior staff.

I nod. 'Hi, Betty.' I reach for her hand. It is ice-cold. 'I'm Christie. I'll get you sitting up on the trolley and we'll go across to A&E. Nothing to worry about, but best to get you checked over. I think I saw you on my way in? In reception?'

'Betty came in to see Patient Liaison this morning, but was early, so she came for a coffee and had a bit of a tight chest. All her obs are fine, but she's had a rough time, haven't you, Betty?'

I notice her expression. Terrified.

'Betty lost her husband to a heart attack recently.'

'I'm very sorry to hear that,' I say, pulling the blanket closer around her. Her temperature is dangerously low. 'How's the pain now?'

She shakes her head. 'I don't want to cause any fuss,' she says. 'It's not bad. Probably something I ate.'

Betty does not look like a patient having a heart attack (myocardial infarction), though older women do not always exhibit the classic signs that you'd expect – chest pain, numbness, tightness, tingling, pins and needles – and occasionally feel no pain at all. Ischaemic heart disease is the most common cause of death in most Western countries, and a major cause of hospital admissions. We see lots of patients suffering heart attacks in hospitals, and many of them are not initially in hospital for that reason. They come for dental appointments or to visit a relative, or to have bloods taken, and the stress of the hospital environment seems to be enough to tip people over the edge. A heart attack is different from a cardiac arrest. A heart attack is caused by atherosclerosis, or hardening of the arteries – a restriction in blood supply to the tissues, and a shortage of oxygen and glucose needed to keep the tissue alive. A cardiac arrest results from the heart stopping entirely, from any cause. But Betty is not sweating or grey, and although her pulse is thready (thin), it feels regular and is palpable.

With help from me and the porter, Betty slowly climbs onto the trolley and I sit her up, wrap as much of the blanket as I can around her thin shoulders, and over her face I put a non-rebreathing oxygen mask – a mask with a pillowy bag at the bottom, which keeps the oxygen concentration levels high. Oxygen is potentially dangerous in the treatment of heart attacks, as it can constrict already-constricted blood vessels. But in medical emergencies where a patient might be critically ill, oxygen is essential. It is also good if you are hungover. But it smells disgusting, it is drying, and having a face-mask placed over you means that you can't see properly and the fear escalates.

I try and reassure Betty. 'This will make you more comfortable.' I walk beside her as the porter pushes the trolley, thinking about how the hospital arteries are much like our own, as the smallest blockage causes us to stop and start until people move aside to let us through.

Arteries and veins have been misunderstood throughout history. In the second century AD, Galen, a Greek biologist and philosopher who practised medicine (he was a surgeon to gladiators), said that 'Throughout the body the animal arteries are mingled with veins, and veins with arteries.' There was a belief that veins contained natural spirits, and arteries contained animal spirits. During medieval times, arteries were thought to contain spiritual blood – the vital spirit. But although our understanding has clearly advanced beyond belief, there is always some truth in history. In studying the arteries, Galen further identified what remains true of arteries (and can be applied metaphorically to hospitals) today: 'It is a useful thing for all parts of the animal to be nourished'.

Tucked down the corridor to the right of us is the hospital cinema, showing the latest films for patients and relatives (and apparently staff, though I've never known any staff member with the time to go there), with a special chair for the nurse, paid for by a charity, who is on hand for reassurance or to deal with emergencies. Next to that is the sexual-health clinic (always busy, standing room only). Betty and I carry on, past the ambulatory medical unit, where a crowd is gathered around a man using a wheelchair who has an unlit cigarette in his mouth and another behind his ear, and is swearing loudly. There is a drip-stand with a large cylinder of frothy clear fluid hanging behind him, running into a thin white tube that eventually burrows into the top of his chest like a misplaced umbilical cord.

'Nearly there,' I say.

These people, the chaos: the spiritual blood of the hospital. The branch- and twig-like arteries and veins leading towards the centre: A&E.

A&E is frightening. It reminds us that life is fragile – and what could be more frightening than that? A&E teaches us that we are vulnerable and, despite our best efforts, we can't predict who will trip on a pavement, causing a catastrophic bleed to the brain; whose roof will collapse, leading to the traumatic amputation of a limb, a broken neck, a broken back, bleeding to death; who will be part of a couple married for sixty years until the wife's dementia results in her injuring her husband. Or who will be in the wrong place at the wrong time: a man with a knife plunged into his heart by a teenage gang member; or a woman beaten and kicked in her pregnant stomach.

There is beauty in A&E, too: a togetherness, where all conflict is forgotten. There is no sleepwalking through the day, as an A&E nurse. Every day is intensely felt and examined, and truly lived. But my hand always shakes when I push open the door – even now, after many years as a nurse. I've never worked solely in A&E, although I spend a lot of time there, in my job as a resuscitation officer. Nursing requires fluidity, being able to adapt and push energy in the direction where patients and colleagues need you, even if it is unfamiliar. Still, A&E scares me. Unlike the staff in the canteen who put out the call for Betty, the staff in A&E only put out a 2222 crash call to the resuscitation team if things are desperate, or if a trauma arrives that requires specialist doctors.

A&E is unpredictable. There are some traffic patterns though. During the week, the mornings are for mothers who have nursed their babies all night and, in the cold light of day, realise they are worse, not better. Daytimes are for accidents and injuries, and the evenings are for office workers who can't get a GP appointment and don't want to take time off work.

Anything can happen on weekday nights, and people tend to come to A&E at night only if they are truly sick. Yet from Thursday evening through to Monday morning party-people fill the corridors, wild-eyed and twitching; there is a steady stream on Sunday mornings, and the later in the day they arrive, the sicker they are: young men and women who have been taking all manner of amphetamines, their pupils as big as the moon, or the alcoholic heroin users with eyes as small as pinpricks, not seeing, not letting in light.

A&E is full of police, shouting relatives, patients lined up with flimsy curtains separating them; an elderly person having a stroke next to an alcoholic, next to a pregnant woman with high blood pressure, next to a carpenter with a hand injury, next to a patient with first-presentation multiple sclerosis, next to a young person suffering from sickle-cell crisis or a child with sepsis. Heart attacks, brain aneurisms, strokes, pneumonia, diabetic ketoacidosis, encephalitis, malaria, asthma, liver failure, kidney stones, ectopic pregnancies, burns, assaults and mental-health crises ... dog-bitten, broken-boned, respiratory-failing, seizing, drug-overdosing, horse-kicked, mentally ill, impaled, shot and stabbed. Once, a head half-sawn off.

Betty's face is grimacing. She reaches out for my hand as we walk through the large waiting area, the patients sitting on plastic chairs or standing lined up against the walls, leaning on the posters. Nobody looks at her. It's as if they see right through her. She is invisible. I read the posters as we pass:

If you have been vomiting or had diarrhoea in the last 48 hours, please tell the unit manager.

If you are aged 12–50 tell the radiographer if you might be pregnant.

Hurt yourself? Injured? Seizure? Call NHS Direct. Chest pain? Not breathing? Call 999.

There's a sink next to the posters. Two containers screwed onto the wall. One contains hand-wash. The other is empty: the alcohol gel has long since been removed. Alcoholics would come into the hospital and drink the hand-gel to get to its alcohol content. Those desperate enough to do that obviously need help but, at bursting point, the only strategy often available is to remove the gel. Nobody has time to scoop up a homeless alcoholic from underneath a sink and deliver treatment for whatever damage they have already done to their system. Bleeding oesophageal varices, as a result of cirrhosis of the liver, is one of the most distressing things I've ever seen – the bursting of blood veins inside the throat, until blood is spewing out. And, as with all complications of alcohol dependency, it can be a consequence of less alcohol than you'd imagine.

Most of the patients sitting on the small chairs at the side of us have someone with them. Arguments have been forgotten;

hands are being held, hair stroked. A few patients are crying. I think of Hogarth's portrayal of London in the painting *Gin Lane* when looking at the hospital waiting area. The poverty is palpable. There are drunk mothers and skeletal fathers. The room smells of body odour and of the metal of old blood. Accident and Emergency may not have changed as much as you might initially think since 1215, when the nuns and monks running a London hospital saw it as a place to provide shelter for the poor, sick and homeless. The first nurses at one such hospital began training on 9th July 1860 and, upon graduation, would be given a chance to visit Florence Nightingale in her own home – an exciting occasion for a few people to meet her in person, but also terrifying: Nightingale kept notes on the students in the school, including their 'character'. What would she make of me?

The hospital remained a place for the poor throughout the nineteenth century, though nursing was becoming formalised by then. Nursing carries with it the echoes of history: nurses would have lost their jobs, had they married. There are, of course, plenty of married nurses now; and, as a junior nurse, I knew a large group of unmarried matrons in the profession, some of whom were living in Spencer House nurses' home, a place we referred to as 'Spinster House', as we failed to imagine how much of a person good nursing requires. Nursing is a career that demands a chunk of your soul on a daily basis. The emotional energy needed to care for people at their most vulnerable is not limitless and there have been many days when, like most nurses, I have felt spent, devoid of any further capacity to give. I feel lucky that my family and friends are forgiving.

Betty coughs, puts her hand over her mouth. Her thin shoulders shake. She reaches for the handbag that I've put at the end of the bed. I lift it higher onto her lap and she gets out a crumpled tissue, wipes her mouth and puts it back in the bag. She keeps hold of the bag, clutching it as if it's a child. I put my hand on her arm, 'Nearly there.'

We pass the door to the outside area, where there's a queue of ambulances: a doctor nips in and out to treat people who are waiting, while they still lie on the hard ambulance trolleys, and apologises for the lack of beds. There is a cleaner constantly mopping the floors, and occasionally she shouts into the air above her head: she has a long-standing mental illness, and the NHS is a non-judgemental employer. The staff come from every possible country, every background, and completely reflect the patients they serve. I've worked with nurses from all corners of the world; nurses who've been homeless themselves; one who worked as an escort to support her studies; nurses who have family members who are dying or who are themselves going through cancer; those who are caring, outside the work environment, for young children and elderly relatives; nurses who are gay, straight, non-binary, transgendered; who are refugees; who are from incredibly wealthy backgrounds or from the kind of council estates where police only travel in groups. Surely there are very few professions with such a diverse cast of characters.

There is movement in nursing, between wards and specialities, and in London there's a high turnover of staff moving between hospitals, but in other parts of the UK nurses tend to stay longer and put down permanent roots. 'I'll have to wait for someone to retire or die, if I want a promotion,' a friend moving to rural Cumbria tells me. But regardless of where the hospital is located, there is an army of people staffing the NHS to meet the needs of the masses: such as the women who make clothes for babies or work in the shop; the kitchen staff; the women from the linen room; the pharmacy assistants; the biomedical engineers.

Dozens of different languages and accents are spoken in A&E, and the list of interpreters behind the receptionist's desk is ever-growing. It rarely gets used. People often have a young relative with them, or there is a porter or cleaner from that particular part of the world. There are arguments against translation from non-experts; a suspicion, on the part of the nurses and doctors, that the words are being softened and not translated precisely, but it's quicker than finding an interpreter.

I wheel Betty on, past the separate children's A&E, the line of beds where there is a long rectangular desk, at the side of which lie piles of paperwork: Do Not Resuscitate forms, observation charts, admission notes. There are shelves and glass doors behind which are cupboards full of equipment, laid out on large pull-out trays; and in front of the doors there are crash trolleys equipped with everything that might be needed, if someone has a cardiac arrest. Betty looks all around her, her head flicking from side to side. She holds her bag tight to her chest. Still, everyone we pass looks at me, and not at Betty. She remains invisible.

At the end of the resuscitation area there is a man on a trolley and two paramedics next to him, a prison officer beside them. There are police, too – but standing at the nurses' station, so they could be unrelated. 'We retrieved some items from the patient's person,' a paramedic once told me. 'We've double-bagged them.' Paramedics have an interesting way of speaking, using language in a slightly formal way, even when off-duty. I often wonder if this is to prevent them from laughing out loud, or crying or retching as they hand over. When I asked what she meant by 'double-bagged them', she said they were contaminated. 'He'd put them up his bum. The mobile phone. And the charger.'

There is a trauma team wearing tabards (a kind of apron) surrounding the next patient: Lead Consultant, Nurse One, Anaesthetist, Orthopaedic Surgeon, Nurse Two. I push Betty to one side. 'I'll leave you here for a minute with the porter, Jamie, okay? Be right back.'

Sandra, the nurse in charge of A&E, is easy to spot. She looks the most harassed and is walking quickly, eyes scanning everywhere. I am not sure why doctors and nurses end up working in A&E, but they are usually adrenaline-junkies. They are fit and unafraid, and they think on their feet, with a no-nonsense kind of intelligence. All the A&E nurses I know are incredibly sarcastic, though I'm not sure if this is a prerequisite for working there.

Sandra stops in front of a bed space where a large number of nurses and doctors are crowding around a patient who is crying.

I walk over. 'Hi, Sandra. I've got a patient, Betty – crash call to the canteen and she has chest pain. Where do you want her?'

Sandra nods at me. 'We're full. Obvs. But get her in bed space one for now?'

I glance at Betty, who is on the other side of the room, still holding her bag. The porter is chatting to her, though, and she has her eyes open. I'm glad she is not looking in this direction.

'Stabbed in three places,' Sandra says, her head nodding towards the crying sound. 'I haven't stopped all night.'

It occurs to me that she is on a night shift from the night before: fourteen hours so far on her feet. People wonder how nurses afford to live in London, but the truth is that they don't. Like Sandra, most of them travel in from outside the city, adding two or three hours to their twelve-and-a-half-hour night shift.

Two nurses are checking details on small packets of red blood cells. Another nurse has already stuck defibrillator pads to the patient's chest and is allocating tasks.

Sandra swoops forward to the stabbing victim as the machines start to alarm in front of her. I leave the bed space. 'Bed one,' she repeats.

The porter helps me slide Betty's trolley down to the other end of the cubicles.

We walk past a patient who is thrashing around and looks likely to hurt herself: she's on a makeshift bed, a safe place of pillows on the floor, until she can be nursed in a room with no sharp edges or items to cause harm. There is a special room in A&E for patients with mental-health problems, although it's inevitably full. Patients who are suffering from severe mental-health disorders have an unacceptable wait in Accident and Emergency – a patient can wait twelve hours, or even longer, and the environment of A&E is completely inappropriate for patients who are already vulnerable and disorientated.

The psychiatric liaison nurse in A&E is covered with tattoos and wears DM boots with frayed laces. She has an increasingly difficult job. The level of responsibility is over-whelming, and the system is failing. But still the psychiatric nurse has to be calm at all times. This patient is clearly very distressed and is punching the air, and the nurse is sitting on the floor next to her, talking in a soft, low voice. I wonder how many hours she'll be sitting there, occasionally being attacked, kicked and hit. According to NICE, the number of reported assaults against NHS staff in one year was 68,683, and 69 per cent occurred in mental-health settings. The word 'reported' is telling. Violence and aggression towards hospital staff is estimated to cost the NHS £69 million a year. What would happen if every nurse reported every incident? The nurse sitting on the floor will not be reporting the hours that she spends today being hit. She'll sit with the patient and will not judge, and she will ignore a couple of bruises.

'Look at that poor nurse,' says Betty as we push past. 'They don't pay you girls enough.'

We leave the resuscitation area, past the cubicles of A&E where Sandra is still busy, and go through to the Majors area, passing a line of patients on trolleys in the corridor, waiting to go to wards. They are all seriously ill and require a hospital bed, but there's no room on the wards; or they are waiting to be seen, having been triaged – assessed for the severity of their illness – and needing to be processed in four hours, although on days like this they can wait much, much longer. Or die, unnoticed, on trolleys.

The porter wheels Betty into the empty bed space, which is being cleaned. A nurse I don't recognise smiles at me as she wipes down the bed, chair, monitor and trolley. There is a whiteboard on the wall, and next to it a sink with a pack of gloves and space for a roll of aprons. Above the sink there's handwash and Hibiscrub, to minimise the risk of infection, and a gap where the alcohol gel used to be. I put on an apron, then help Betty slide over onto the bed. The nurse rushes off before I can say anything. 'I'll get the twelve-lead,' she says.

Betty is getting worse. Her face looks concave and she is shivering, her teeth chattering. She is the colour of the sheet behind her head, it looks as though she is disappearing into a cloud.

I tuck the blanket around her, careful to move slowly: her skin is paper-thin and she has bruises at different stages patterning her arms like late-summer roses. The blanket is blue and a bit scratchy, but she is still shivering.

I check her temperature again, using a small machine that sits just inside her ear and beeps when it's ready. Betty's skin does not feel as cold now, but the elderly have means of disguising problems with their temperature. Sometimes a very low – rather than very high – temperature in elderly patients can indicate sepsis: a life-threatening infection. I've always been fascinated by temperature, and the tiny margin within which our bodies can operate. To maintain life we have to keep our core temperature within fairly tight parameters. But we can survive well in the freezing cold; patients who almost drown in winter shut their own brains down so effectively that it becomes a protective mechanism. The other extreme is malignant hyperthermia which can happen as a rare reaction to anaesthetic drugs, causing a rise in temperature until someone's brain is cooking on the inside.

Betty's temperature is not extreme, but it's still dangerously low. She's been at home, with no heating, I suspect. There are millions of people in the UK living in fuel poverty, who cannot pay their heating bills.

'Betty, I'm going to get you a bear-hugger. It blows hot air over you and warms you up a bit. It's very cosy. The other nurse is bringing a machine that measures your heart, to check everything is okay.'

'Thank you, love. I'm all right, though. I don't want to be a nuisance. I can see how busy you are. I know the heart machine...'

'You're not a nuisance at all. That's what we're here for.' I smile at her and take her hand, giving it a gentle squeeze. 'Now, can I get you a sandwich and cup of tea?'

Betty smiles. 'You're so kind,' she says.

'I'll see what I can rustle up.'

I find the bear-hugger next to a cubicle where a nurse pokes his head out from behind a curtain and smiles at me. 'You don't see this anywhere else,' he says.

'The girl in bed five is fluorescent-yellow,' Francisco, a Spanish nurse I recognise from training, explains, coming over towards us. He stands next to me and waves his hands in the air. 'The colour of neon. So we call the paediatric crash team. In Spain there are no young people in gutters, one shoe on, one shoe off. Here, that's all we deal with. So we think she's a suicide. Liver damage. Paracetamol overdose, you know. We started the treatment, sending bloods for toxicology and all of that. But when she regained consciousness and we questioned her, she laughs. "I'm not suicidal," she says. "It's fake tan."' Francisco disappears to his bed space and draws the curtain abruptly behind him.

I push the machine back to Betty, picking up an egg-and-cress sandwich on the way. The sandwich looks dry and unappealing, its edges curled and uniform. I would love to have cut Betty a thick slice of fresh bread and to have served it with real butter and jam.

When I return, the bedside nurse has already performed the ECG and has left the crescent moon of stickers around Betty's chest.

'They said it looked okay,' she tells me.

I'm not at all surprised. Betty lost her husband to a heart attack, and then she suffered chest pain. Though it's never advisable to jump to conclusions, I'm pretty certain she is experiencing a panic attack.

'Good news,' I say. 'Now to warm you up a bit.' The bear-hugger is made of white billowing paper like fabric and, once over Betty and plugged in, it encloses her in what looks like a miniature hot-air balloon. Her temperature should increase by a degree an hour, and her blood sugar, which is also low – no doubt from lack of eating – should rise to normal levels after the sandwich and sweet tea. Finding an extension and a plug socket isn't easy, so I do some shifting around of chairs and equipment, and of Betty. Finally, the bear-hugger is on.

'It *is* like having a hug,' she says. She starts looking better almost immediately. She holds the ring on the chain around her neck.

'A bear-hugger is exactly that. I'm going to leave you to get some rest now, Betty, and the nurse will be back in a while. Okay?'

She nods. Half-smiles. 'This material,' she says, 'reminds me of my wedding dress.'

I look at the bear-hugger, then at Betty's eyes. They have filled with light. I pause. Betty is not sick; she does not have thickened arteries, requiring surgery and drugs and technology. But she does need something. Something nurses can give. I pick up her hand again, the warmth of the machine making both of us exactly the same temperature. It is hard to tell for a second where my hand stops and hers begins.

'We had no way of getting material,' she says. 'But we did have parachute silk. We had egg-and-cress sandwiches then, too. I remember the taste. And coronation chicken, though Stan picked out all the raisins. Never ate any fruit or vegetables, did my Stan.' She laughs. 'I used to try and sneak them into his beef stew, you know – mash up some carrots and swede. But he always knew. He'd pretend to choke and ask me to hit him on the back. Silly old fool.'

If a couple have been married for a lifetime, it often happens that when one dies, the other dies soon afterwards. We can't write 'Broken-hearted' on the cause-of-death forms, of course, but that's what I believe it to be. Broken-hearted people stop taking care of themselves. They don't eat, wash, sleep. They are between worlds, cold with grief.

I discover that Betty has no family to rally round her, like my nan did after my granddad died, to make sure that she eats meals and has comforting hugs, and keeps warm, and to give her sleeping tablets and soup. There is a physiological response to grief, and the sweet tea that is offered when someone is in a state of shock actually helps the patient's blood sugar rise to a non-dangerous level. Sweet tea can prevent seizure, coma, even death, and people's blood sugar drops in response to serious illness, grief or shock more often than you would imagine. It is not necessarily related to diabetes at all, and is easy to fix; but, if missed, it can be disastrous.

Betty is completely alone in her flat now, which explains her state of health and her chest pain, more than any machine can. And the way she wolfs her dry sandwich down in gulps. Her colour improves as she speaks, and she becomes more alert and sits up a bit. I stand listening to her, holding her paper-thin hand, which is almost as crumpled as the fabric around her; it shakes less and less as she talks, until it is steady and warmer.

I can't stay for long. There is another patient's angry relative a few curtains down, who is staring at me, pacing up and down slightly. I need to run back to the resuscitation office and fill in the audit form, and get a proper handover. There's teaching to organise and kit to check, and my boss will be wondering where on earth I am – he's already commented that I move in mysterious ways. There's too much to do.

But I stay another minute, and close my eyes for a while and listen. Betty has a wonderful story. And if I listen hard enough, I stop seeing a frail old woman alone on a hospital trolley, and instead watch a young woman in a dress made from parachute silk, dancing with her new husband, Stan.

2

Everything You Can Imagine
is Real

Kindness is the language which the deaf can hear and the blind can see.

Mark Twain

It turns out my route into nursing is a combination of many influential experiences. I am fifteen when I arrive home from school to find our living room filled with adults with Down's syndrome and other disabilities. One of them, a middle-aged obese woman wearing a neon-pink crop top, is sitting squashed next to my dad, saying, 'I love you.' My dad has his glasses pushed up close on his face and is wearing a terrified expression. A man standing next to them is laughing loudly, while another woman is rocking back and forth, making incomprehensible sounds. I have many questions. But before I can ask anything, my mum arrives carrying my brother's *Star Wars* tray, on which is a jug of orange squash, cups and a pack of custard creams.

My mum, at this point, is training to be a social worker and is on a placement in a residential group home for people

with severe learning disabilities, some of them with challenging behaviour. She is, I suspect, becoming a communist.
This is causing some difficulties with my conservative dad,
who is now getting redder and redder and is trying to move
away from the woman, who is saying 'I love you' on repeat,
like a broken toy.

'Oh, Natasha,' my mum says. 'Leave him alone. My poor
husband can barely breathe!'

'Erm... What's going on?' I ask.

Mum hands out the squash. 'Well, we popped in for a cold
drink, but actually we're all going to have dinner together.'

I actually feel my eyebrows move up my forehead. I pray
to any God I can think of that none of my friends decide to
pop round. I am not yet a social liberal.

It turns into a lovely dinner, and it alters my thinking and
misconceptions; by the end of the evening I feel embarrassed
by my lack of understanding of my own privilege and prejudice.
And although I don't realise it at the time, my mum teaches
me much that day about the power balance in care: 'Why
should I know all about their lives, and spend time in people's
private homes, and they not know anything at all about me?
That doesn't seem fair.'

Even my dad, after untangling himself from Natasha and
cooking everyone roast lamb for dinner, enjoys the evening.
When it is time to go, however, Natasha will not get into the
minibus. It takes ages, and a promise of another dinner, before

she will leave my dad's side. 'I'm sorry for loving your husband,' she says to my mum as they finally leave the house.

'That's okay,' she replies. 'I totally understand.'

My dad and I wave them off and stand motionless and wordless for some time, staring at the empty, quiet road.

A year and a bit later, I am following in Mum's footsteps and before nursing training I am working with adults who have moderate to severe learning and/or physical disabilities. I find the work challenging and rewarding.

Anthony has no learning disability, but has been diagnosed with bipolar disorder. I spend many hours in his kitchen helping him with the cooking, helping him to eat, and listening to his stories about how he finally got a diagnosis, after trying to buy thirty mopeds. His speech is severely affected by cerebral palsy, so I have to listen hard and he never once gets frustrated if I ask him to repeat himself. Another resident uses an eye-pointing board, whereby she looks at each letter to spell out a word. This is before the age of decent technology, and although there are many negative associations with the advances in technology, I often think of her – and of others with severe disabilities, whose lives must surely have been transformed by it.

Anthony suffers from constant jerking movements and needs full-time care. His mental health is fragile, despite medication that has evened out his mood. And despite all the challenges he faces, we laugh and laugh and laugh. Anthony's sister often visits and I am always surprised that she, who has no disabilities or mental-health conditions that I know of, seems perpetually miserable. 'She never stops moaning,' comments Anthony, after one visit.

'The nature of happiness is a complicated thing,' I say. And Anthony grins and tells me I'm weird.

We have a strange relationship. He is a fifty-eight-year-old man, and one of my tasks as a sixteen-year-old carer is to help him use the toilet: either lift him out of the wheelchair onto the toilet seat, then wipe him afterwards, or help him pee into a bottle. There are other residents who need similar personal care: the changing of sanitary towels, or rolling on a condom-type sheath attached to a urine bag, for one older man who is incontinent. I can't imagine now how I managed to perform such intimate tasks without embarrassment on both sides. Anthony is severely physically disabled and mentally unwell and some days are harder than others. But I've never met anyone else I've cared for who could make me laugh until drops of tea fall out of my nostrils. *I mean, who needs thirty fucking mopeds?*

There are four distinct training pathways to nursing in the UK: adult nursing, child nursing, mental-health and learning-disability nursing. But none of the branches makes much sense to me: in the same way that you can't split body and mind, I'm not certain that an early specialism in nursing is helpful to either nurse or patient. It is perfectly feasible, for example, that you might be caring for an adolescent who has both learning disabilities and mental-health concerns, and who has also sustained physical injuries in a car accident.

I think carefully about learning-disability nursing, remembering Natasha and how my mum loved her placement working with adults with learning disabilities; how rewarding she found helping someone live independently; and how interesting that disability is concerning the construction of society, as much as anything else. But I opt to train, initially, in mental-health nursing. I am partly thinking of Anthony, but also aiming for minimal exposure to blood. Following my fainting episode on seeing my own blood being taken, I feel incredibly sensitive. Whenever I see blood – even on television – the back of my head seems to float away from me until the room spins. I have to stop reading books if there are descriptions of bloody scenes, or depictions of gruesome murders. It is ludicrous to suddenly develop a phobia, but I am already in too deep and am too proud to admit that nursing might not be the best option for me after all.

Caring for minds sounds as if it would be easier to cope with than caring for bodies. So when I discover that the word 'psychiatry' was identified in 1808 by Johann Christian Reil, a German doctor, and means 'the medical treatment of the soul' (he shared my own belief that advances in civilisation create more madness), my mind is firmly made up.

The terms 'mental-health nurse' and 'psychiatric nurse' are interchangeable now, but the language of nursing has changed. In the eighteenth and nineteenth centuries the term 'keeper' was used to describe nurses working in mental-health settings – reflecting the horrific history of the understanding and treatment of the mentally ill, and the nurse's role as one of control and restriction.

It is finally my first day on the wards, after weeks in college when we have weekly anatomy and physiology exams with the medical students, and long lectures about the nature of nursing, the academic language enough to make all of us sleepy. I've learned about risk models for suicide and self-harm, and dementia-care mapping; about early intervention, harm reduction, classification systems, psycho-pharmacology, care-planning, boundaries, stigma and discrimination, advocacy, power imbalances, law, ethics and consent. I've read lots about the history of mental-health care, which is morbidly fascinating. But sitting in a classroom with my contemporaries feels very distant from being a nurse on a ward.

I wake up at 5 a.m., too nervous to sleep; my stomach is a ball of elastic bands. There is no uniform for mental-health nurses, simply what the lecturer calls 'mufti': smart casual, no jeans. 'Your mufti is slightly too mufti,' one of the lecturers remarks about my wardrobe. I have ID, which takes a whole morning to sort out: following winding basement corridors in the hospital, past the hydrotherapy pool where the smell of chlorine is strong enough to make your eyes water (incontinent patients are not uncommon); through the hospital atrium, past the equipment room, where the staff offer no eye contact and organise large walls of stock, the entire bunker-sized room like the inside of an odds-and-sods drawer. I pass the general hospital labs, where there are double doors and entrance codes, and the staff are pale and intense. 'I spent six months pipetting yeast,' my friend tells me, after swapping her university course from biomedical chemical engineering to business studies. 'Lab work takes a special person – very special.' I walk on, past the queue to the dental floors, a terrifying tower of swollen-faced, doubled-over, crying people who need emergency dentistry. Eventually I find a small room with a large tattoo-covered security guard, who prints the ID and puts it onto a clip-badge. When I see the photo – which is terrible (I am puffing out my cheeks, for some reason, and look like a chipmunk) – I ask him if it would be possible to redo it. He simply lowers his head and stares at me, until I leave the room, walking backwards, nearly knocking over a chair. 'Sorry, sorry,' I say, apologising for whatever I did to cause that look.

I clip the awful photo to my shirt and glance in the mirror, then take a deep breath. I am shaking and I can feel my heart running upwards to my neck. What do I know about anything?

I look at my too-mufti mufti. My T-shirt is crumpled and my trousers are too long, and are frayed at the bottom. I have cut my own hair, in an attempt to save money. I ask the mirror, 'Mirror, mirror, on the wall, who's bricking it the most of all?'

The building at the back of the car park looks much like the nurses' home, but with tiny, dirty white bars criss-crossing the windows. The psychiatric block is simply that: an entire block separate from the rest of the hospital. The first hospitals for curing mental illness were established in India during the third century BC. In the UK, the Bethlem (Bethlem Royal Hospital, known in the past as 'Bedlam') is Europe's oldest psychiatric hospital and has operated continuously for more than 600 years; it currently houses the National Psychosis Unit. Some hospitals have psychiatric wards, or outpatient clinics in the main hospital; and other hospitals, like Bethlem, are purely mental-health specialists. But regardless of the layout, the landscape and the atmosphere are different from the other wards.

I press the door buzzer. After pressing again and a long wait, a woman lets me in and directs me to the lifts, without asking who I am, or looking once at the awful photograph on my ID. The door to the acute admission ward is locked, too, and I have another long wait. Each floor is another sub-speciality, and psychiatry has many: Admission, Female, Male, Mixed, Organic Psychiatry, Older People Psychiatry, Adolescent Suite, Eating Disorder Unit, Drug and Alcohol

Rehabilitation Unit, Psychosis, Forensic Psychiatry, Psycho-logical Medicine, Mother and Baby, ECT (electro-convulsive therapy) Suite.

There's also now a ward for people who have somatic disorders, as in, physical symptoms of emotional distress, such as being unable to walk or becoming incontinent. 'This is increasingly a widespread problem,' says a nurse at the South London and Maudsley NHS Foundation Trust. 'The ward is full of patients who stay in bed for months, unable to walk or use the toilet, without the use of their legs; or who are blind, have constant pain, numbness, seizures. And it turns out there is nothing medically wrong with them. Emotions are that powerful.' Suzanne O'Sullivan, an eminent neurologist and expert in the condition, remains astounded by its frequency. 'Every week I have to tell someone their disability has a psychological cause, a diagnosis that is often angrily rejected.' You cannot separate mind and body. We are all souls, housed in flesh.

By the time I get in and find the staffroom, I'm late. I hadn't figured I would spend twenty minutes waiting. The nurse in charge does not look up. He's writing in a large black diary. 'You've missed handover,' he says. He has a scruffy beard and is wearing jeans. His mufti is beyond 'mufti'.

'I'm sorry. It's my first day.'

He briefly looks at me, then back down. 'Go and find Sue,' he says. 'She's your mentor.'

I stand, unable to move. My stomach is alive and writhing with nerves. The handover room has a filing cabinet, upon which balances a dead spider plant. I focus on the brown curled spikes, soft with age. The table that the nurse leans on is full of coffee-ringed marks and half-drunk coffee; and there's a motorbike helmet covered in stickers, with a small dent in it. The room smells of tuna and tobacco. It is too hot, and there is an industrial-sounding hum coming from the giant radiator. A relentless buzzing.

He looks up again. Smiles. Lets the smile drop quickly. His pen continues to write as his eyes meet mine. 'Sue,' he says. 'Find Sue. She's your mentor. You'll be fine.'

'I'm only seventeen,' I want to say. 'And I fainted during induction week.' Instead, I take a breath and go out to the main ward, past the nurses' station, a small square area separated by sideboards like a kitchen island, and desks; there are locked cupboards against the back, presumably the drugs cupboards. There is a coffee room with people sitting around, and next to that a smoking area outside at the back. Thankfully, most mental-health units have moved a million miles forward since that time, in terms of attitudes, treatments and architecture. But not all of them. And not far enough.

But this is 1994; the smoking area is full. Through the smoke, which is something like that of a late-night jazz club, I can see a dozen people, men and women. The ward stretches out in front of me, with bedrooms on either side. I have no idea where to find Sue, and it is impossible to tell the staff from the patients.

I stand looking at all the patients and staff milling around the ward. I have no idea what I am meant to be doing. 'Sue?' I ask every woman – patient or nurse: who knows? I walk through the ward, past the faded prints on either side of the wall: Dalí, Rembrandt, Van Gogh. The sadness of the prints with no glass covering them, curled up at the corners like old beer mats. I walk past the reading room, devoid of books, where two women sit and stare straight ahead. 'Sue?' I ask, but there is no response. There's a television on loud, showing a daytime programme that nobody is watching. It's a confusing and unpleasant place for me. I can only imagine how it must feel to be forced to live here when you are mentally unwell.

A small woman appears in front of me, carrying a large set of keys. She's wearing jeans and a shirt and has a large smile. 'Are you looking for Sue? You must be the new student.'

I nod, exhale. 'Christie,' I say, offering my clammy hand.

'Well, let's get you settled in, then you can read the notes.' She lowers her voice. 'Always read the notes before you meet the patients.'

Something about her tone makes my nerves creep up into my neck until I feel thumping in my head.

A tall man is pacing the corridor in front of us. 'They are stealing my kidneys, too,' he says. 'Taking them out. And my heart, to switch them over. They put machines in me that record everything. Take slices of heart. Replace the chambers inside it with prisons. They want my liver. And my intestines.'

Sue ignores him. 'Derek!' she says. He walks away and into a bedroom. A slamming door brings another woman out of a room to our left and she looks left and right, before following Derek into his bedroom. I stare until Sue holds up the keys and shakes them in front of my face. 'Staffroom, always locked; and the medicine cupboard. Always lock the stationery cupboard, too; there is equipment in there that could cause harm.' I follow her, trying to take in her every word. 'And people nick things. It's an acute admissions ward,' she says, 'so we get a mixed bag of people: schizophrenics, psychotics, depressives, borderline personality disorders.' She lowers her voice, leans in towards me. 'If you believe such a thing exists. Anyhow, you just met Derek. He was admitted last night. He stopped taking his meds, as you can see. There's an elderly care unit upstairs, where they see patients with organic diseases and associated mental-health problems. The psychopaths, personality disorders and criminal mental-health problems are usually found in the forensic units,' she smiles, 'but not always.'

I follow Sue around the ward as she waves her arm in each direction. I think of all the psychiatric disorders that could lead to an acute admission, for assessment of the kind I know they perform on this ward. It's an open ward, despite the number of keys and locked doors, which means that people can leave at any point, although I know some of the patients will be held under a section of the Mental Health Act – for up to six months, in certain cases. A community psychiatric-nurse friend relays stories about sectioning vulnerable people. 'It's sometimes a nurse's responsibility, if they've done the appropriate training and are an approved mental-health professional, to order a deprivation of liberty and send a patient to hospital.'

The ethics of compulsory admissions to mental-health wards have kept me awake on many nights: the Mental Capacity Act and the Mental Health Act, which form the law that gives a nurse a legal framework to make decisions on the patient's behalf. The idea of a nurse as a 'keeper' is a horrific one. The five principles of the Mental Capacity Act acknowledge that before a judgement is made, the nurse must consider whether the decision can be achieved in a way to minimise the restriction of a patient's rights and freedom. But the ability to remove a person's freedom feels an enormous and dangerous responsibility to lay, initially at least, on just one person. Luckily, I tell myself that I am years away from that level of training. Even so, there is a strange imbalance in knowing that I can leave, but some of the people I am caring for are too ill to go home. I feel a huge responsibility to get things right.

'Staff toilets,' Sue says. 'Craft room.' I follow her arm towards where two young women and an older man sit around a small table doing some sort of craftwork. 'Anorexics,' Sue says, 'you need to watch them. We did an admission search recently on her,' she points her head at a woman wearing a hoodie. 'She told us she had nothing on her person that was contraband. And then she gave the nurse in charge five razor blades that she'd hidden and said, "You missed those." She had no intention of hurting herself, just wanted to cause trouble for that admitting nurse.'

The two women look strange, and it's hard not to stare: they are rib-winged and feather-boned. I press my teeth together to stop my mouth opening. How awful for someone suffering to see someone else staring, especially a nurse. I have a neighbour who is clearly ill; her bones look as if they might snap when she runs and runs every morning. I always say hello to her, and try and force my eyes not to stare, just like now, though I find it difficult. I wonder if she – like these women – might die. Anorexia remains one of the leading causes of mental-health-related deaths. And it is on the increase. And now 'orthorexia' has arrived: an excessive preoc-cupation with eating healthy food. Orthorexia is not yet listed as an eating disorder by the American Psychiatric Association in the *DSM* (the book of all things related to mental health – the *Diagnostic and Statistical Manual of Mental Disorders*), but I'm pretty sure it will be. Fast forward to an age of Insta-gram and other social media and impossible-to-achieve perfection, and eating disorders such as these will no doubt increase year-on-year. 'These girls are all the super-selective high-achievers. We see so many,' a child and adolescent mental-health nurse comments. 'Anorexia affects girls usually, but boys with eating disorders have risen by twenty-seven per cent in the last three years: double the rate of increase in girls. What a time to be a teenager! The pressure is too much.'

We walk to the other end of the ward. 'Sitting room,' Sue says. A few people are drinking cups of tea, and the TV is droning out another daytime programme that nobody is looking at. 'Art therapy at ten usually pulls in a crowd. Music at one – usually only Keith, as he refuses to wash. Then group therapy, which is voluntary, but we try and drag people along.' Sue smiles. 'All clear?'

I nod. 'Thank you.' But I have no clue what I'm meant to do. What is my role here as a nurse? Do I simply sit with the patients, or try and talk to them, or watch them? Do I learn about the drugs dished out from behind the hatch and their side-effects, or do I attempt to make pottery? Do I encourage the girls suffering from anorexia to eat? Or simply monitor what they are eating? The Royal College of Nursing, in its 'Standards for Pre-Registration' document, states that 'mental-health nurses must use different methods of engaging people, and work in a way that promotes positive relationships focused on social inclusion, human rights and recovery; that is, a person's ability to live a self-directed life, with or without symptoms, that they believe is meaningful and satisfying.'

I like the idea that I can help provide meaning to another person's life, and during the same process search for meaning in my own. But I have no idea how to go about it.

'No problem,' Sue says. 'After lunch the meds kick in, so everyone's usually monged out until the evening, then it's *EastEnders* and a film. No horror, obviously. Or aliens. Especially now Derek is back. He believes he's been abducted and had his kidneys removed by extraterrestrials.' She shakes her head. 'Never tell him he's wrong. I mean, who are we to say that aliens didn't abduct him? Or aren't trying to, anyway. The universe is bigger than we can understand. We don't have proof. But never tell him he's right, either. Also, Pam prefers *Coronation Street*, and we don't want her to get suicidal again.'

'Monged out?' I notice the girls who are clearly suffering with anorexia are looking at me and laughing. 'Suicidal?'

'The meds. Chemical straitjackets. And who's to say that my reality is somehow more real than Derek's? Aliens could be real. It's not our job to disprove. We are not here to dispute the possibility of extraterrestrial activity in another galaxy.' She laughs, a short burst of cackling.

My stomach feels heavier, my mouth fizzes. I feel the back of my head shrinking.

'Of course,' Sue leans towards me and whispers, 'the patients don't know that the medication is full of arsenic. So you mustn't tell them, okay? They put kryptonite in the water here, too. Don't drink anything.'

I turn my head slowly, look at Sue's face and her far-away eyes. 'You're not Sue, are you?'

She laughs again and does a sort of jig from side to side. 'Had you – had you! Sue's on a break.'

I stand still for a few seconds, the heat creeping up my neck and into my face, my cheeks so hot that I can imagine their redness. I feel stupid. The ground wobbles beneath me. I try and remember everything she has told me. It all seems like nonsense already. I have clearly watched too many films. Did I tell her anything? Have I broken any rules already? Will I lose my registration before I even get it? I look at her face. Her eyes meet mine. She holds her chuckling stomach. And then I can't help but join in the laughter with her. My own laughter sings with hers.

She is not Sue, as it turns out, but a woman named Hayley. Despite feeling stupid and a bit terrified, I begin to talk and laugh with her from that day, and every day during my placement Hayley tells me (and anyone else she can) the story of my first day. 'Of course there's no distinction between patients and staff. We can all get ill, and we probably all will, at some stage. Mental illness is no different from having asthma, or a broken bone. So don't worry about it. Why should I not be Sue?' And then she tells me about arsenic, and how the other nurses are not nurses at all, but are sent by the government to control her mind. Hayley is clearly ill, but she teaches me so many things.

The earliest psychiatric nurses were known as 'soul friends', each being matched with a patient to develop a therapeutic relationship, based on friendship. This is back in fashion now, with hospitals hiring people who have personal experience of mental illness to work in recovery colleges – centres around the country that take an educational, rather than clinical, approach to working with people who are suffering from mental illness. I am glad to be matched with Hayley. She makes me laugh, like Anthony used to. I once hear her tell her husband to stop calling her every day: 'I'm having a break,' she says. 'A psychotic break. I'll be home in six months.'

Sue, my mentor (the real one), is a woman from Skegness who has nicotine-stained fingers and bright-purple eyeshadow – and no bunch of keys. She laughs and laughs when I tell her about Hayley. 'Come on now,' she says, 'we've all had a first day. At least I didn't send you for a long weight!'

I follow Sue (after glancing at the ID clipped to her top) to the clinical room, where she and another nurse stock-check the controlled drugs. Pharmacology has made extensive leaps since the late nineteenth century, when a number of sedative drugs were given to patients with a view to chemically restraining them rather than treating their disease. Chloral hydrate is highly addictive (and is sometimes now used as a date-rape drug) and has unpleasant side-effects, and although it is no longer used in mental-health settings, until very recently it was routinely administered in paediatric intensive-care settings to keep children still.

Sue talks continually. 'Drugs don't actually treat disease, in fact they only help with the symptoms. And they are still used to restrain people. We have excellent doctors here, but it's important to remind them that the patient's choice is paramount with regard to their medication, and even whether they choose to take it – if they're not sectioned, that is. This is where the service-users queue up to get their medication in the morning, then lunchtime and evenings. Most of them are fine, but some need lots of encouragement and support.' She speaks the smell of cigarette smoke. 'You have to prep all the charts, and make sure the doctors haven't prescribed the wrong dose. Then we have the morning meeting, which you should go to. Talk about each service-user, any issues, plan and all that. Then it's a ton of paperwork to do with assessments, tribunals, progress notes. Don't look so worried. It will all make sense as we go along.'

If the drugs only alleviate the symptoms, then what does treat the disease? Dr Drake, a professor of community psychiatry in America, says that 'The only effective thing in the psychiatrist's toolkit is helping people succeed in paid employment.' Sue teaches me much about what may, or may not, work in mental-health care. Student nurses on placement are each allocated a mentor who supervises, supports and assesses the student. Occasionally student nurses might spend time with other members of the mental-health team: art psychotherapists, psychologists, social workers and occupational therapists; but most of their time will be with a nurse mentor.

It is a completely hit-and-miss arrangement and, as with anything, some mentors are kind and understanding that a student nurse like me might be terrified, young and naive, while other mentors seem to enjoy the sense of power they have over the student – the hierarchy. I am lucky. Sue is warm and keeps putting her hand on my arm, squeezing gently. 'You'll be grand. Why don't you do a set of obs on Derek? You met him already. He needs physical obs on his charts: blood pressure and all of that.'

I exhale. I have been practising physical observations and feel comfortable with that, in a way I do not yet with other aspects of mental-health nursing: facilitating activities and therapeutic group work beyond my understanding. Filling in charts with temperatures and diet, and fluids and respiratory rates, is a practical and fairly easy task that I feel ready to master. I smile for the first time, feel my jaw unclench and walk towards Derek's room.

Derek is six foot two and has a loud voice that you can hear from outside the hospital. He has been transferred via the Psychiatric Intensive-Care Unit (PICU; not to be confused with the *Paediatric* Intensive-Care Unit, also known as PICU). There he was looked after by tiny female Filipino nurses, who I discover often work in PICU with huge six-foot-plus men, sometimes those who have been self-medicating with drugs and alcohol; they are often very ill and can be violent, but the Filipino nurses tell me they are far less likely to be attacked than their male nurse counterparts. 'The service-users don't feel so threatened, so they are not afraid. And much of the illness is driven by fear. The male nurses have to call us sometimes if they have a very violent or aggressive service-user, so that we can come and calm them down.'

Derek does not seem afraid. But there's a thick Bible on his pillow and he reaches a hand and touches it when I go in.

'Hi, I'm Christie,' I say as I go into his room. It is entirely functional, with a built-in wardrobe, a chest of drawers, a bed and a chair.

Another man sits on a chair opposite him. 'Hi, I'm Vik, one of the psychiatry doctors.' He stands and I shake his hand.

Derek does not stand but nods at me.

'Hi, Derek. I have to take your blood pressure – is that okay?' I see the machine outside the door and reach out an arm to pull it in.

'No,' he says.

Vik sits back down. 'Derek, Christie is here to help. She wants to check you over physically, like we do every day. Quick checks: your blood pressure was slightly raised last night.'

Without any warning, Derek stands up and clenches his fists. He shouts and screams, 'They are trying to steal me. Take my soul out through my nostril or my eye-holes. They're going to eat my eyes and suck the brain through my skull, and drill a hole into my neck, and push a coat hanger up through my throat and hook clumps of it, pull it out, until the rest of my brains fall down. Then they will alter the neurons. Reprogramme me. Put acid on my brain cells and melt them. When they put my brain back inside me, I will be one of them…'

Vik remains sitting. 'Okay, Derek, you're safe. I'm here.' He nods at the door and I walk out slowly, as others rush in. I stand in the doorway as they suddenly surround Derek, who is now shouting louder and louder. I feel tears fill my eyes and course down my face. I have made him worse, not better. I must have said something wrong, or done something wrong. He was fine before I went in.

Sue laughs. 'It's not you. Derek's really unwell, and unfortunately he's unpredictable, like all of our patients. Vik is great, but sometimes we can't de-escalate the situation and have to restrain and sedate people.' She passes me a cup of tea. 'Poor Derek. He's been attacked repeatedly in the community. It's the mentally ill who are in danger from society. Not the other way around.' We are in the staffroom, where I saw the mufti man from handover. I am only halfway through my shift, but I feel exhausted – a sponge wrung out, spaced out and foggy. 'You should write it down. Reflective practice is part of the job. Every day, reflect on what's happened and, if you can, write it down.'

We have completed a module on the critical side of reflective practice, but it's the first time I consider it relevant. Sue is right, of course. Reflective practice – like all nursing theories – has a number of different models and ideas, but essentially it is the process of making sense of real events. It is widely regarded as some kind of emotional protection for nurses who are paying the cost of caring for vulnerable people, and it helps the nurse to understand her own personality, life story and memories and how they influence events. One of the models of reflective practice, developed by Beverley Taylor, a nurse and midwife, acknowledges that 'some questions may remain puzzles'. But I can see Sue's point; finding the meaning in the questions will help. Why did Derek react that way? Why has it upset me so much?

'Keeping a reflective journal helps me stay well,' Sue says, 'and on difficult days I still do it. And you will see how far you're coming, as you move through your placements. That, plus a large gin and tonic at the end of the day…'

Derek isn't the only black man on the unit diagnosed with schizophrenia, which is a serious illness that affects the way a person thinks. Schizophrenia has nothing to do with split or multiple personalities. A friend who suffers from schizophrenia describes it as 'seeing the world in fragments. Trying to make things fit together. But of course one size doesn't fit all, and my experience is completely different from everyone else's.'

There are some commonalities on the Psychiatric Intensive-Care Unit, though. Every single patient at that time is BAME (black, Asian or minority ethnic) and most are from working-class backgrounds. They are displaying – as far as I can see – no more agitated behaviour than Pam, the middle-class white woman who has never been moved to the Intensive-Care Unit. And although I am remembering events from a point twenty years later, the same story exists today. The Mental Health Act, written all those years ago, does not creatively assess cultural and racial stereotypes within society at large. The French philosopher Michel Foucault insisted that madness depends on the society in which it exists, and that cultural, intellectual and economic structures in society construct its experience of madness. There is much work still to be done to explore this. The UK-based AESOP study, which was conducted over a two-year period in three British sites simultaneously (London, Nottingham and Bristol), was the largest to date to conduct a first-contact case-control analysis of psychosis. It found that rates of schizophrenia were markedly elevated in both African-Caribbean and black African people, in both sexes and across all age groups. Afro-Caribbean men are much more likely to receive such a diagnosis. Since the 1960s there have been numerous studies comparing rates of schizophrenia and other psychoses, and all reported incidence rates are significantly higher for black men, with a range from two to eighteen times. A recent report warned about the poor level of service given to black African and Caribbean men, and stated that this group is on average detained five times longer in secure care than other groups. There are no clear answers as to why this happens, although racism at both an individual and institutional level clearly remains a key issue.

I think about what this means for Derek, and what my role is, as a mental-health nurse, to challenge such inequalities. The Royal College of Nursing insists that challenging the inequalities and discrimination that may arise from, or contribute to, mental-health problems is a key responsibility of a mental-health nurse. Human-rights law underpins all aspects of mental-health nursing. But the social and political context of mental health is dirty bath-water. So much of mental-health care happens in the community, and chronic under-funding and cuts to services such as housing and benefits are having a damning effect on our nation's mental health and are, I would imagine, contributing to rising suicide rates. There are many layers of unpleasant truths that health professionals still have trouble expressing, or even acknowledging at times, and which directly contribute to mental-health disorders.

I have always noticed things in London: the queue of almost entirely black people on their way to work, waiting for the bus much too early in the morning. I sit in McDonald's, or the gym, or the British Library, and watch who is cleaning. I notice that the healthcare assistants are black, and the managers of the hospital are white. I notice, too, the brightly coloured elaborate dream-catchers in the dirtiest of windows on south London estates. Working with Derek I begin to think about the higher rates of diagnosis for black men suffering from schizophrenia, and how multi-layered the statistics. I start to reflect.

I am allocated to spend time with Derek regularly and, gradually, I see him improve. He lets me take his blood pressure without any issues and Vik tells me that Derek is to be allowed out on day-release – something Vik calls 'positive risk-taking'. Derek is certainly calmer now, and more able to articulate what he is feeling. As the psychosis becomes less fierce, his character is revealed. He is interested in art and chess during his calm moments, and he tries, and fails, to teach me about both, laughing at me calling the chess pawns 'prawns'. He has an antique chess-board that smells of the sea and tells me it's journeyed around the world for centuries. I am wide-eyed. I discover that he's been eating Scampi Fries, and the smell is on his fingertips, and he laughs again until his face is wet. He teaches me about Frida Kahlo, quoting her regularly: 'They thought I was a Surrealist, but I wasn't. I never painted dreams. I painted my own reality.'

'She understood, you know?' Derek says to me. 'I mean, she really understood reality? "I'm not painting dreams." Do you understand?'

'Sort of,' I say. And I do, sort of. I am beginning to understand what mental-health nursing is, though it is difficult to define. 'A mental-health nurse is a dream-catcher in a desperate window,' I say.

And Derek gives me a look that suggests I've said something either extremely accurate or completely nonsensical.

'It is a constant weighing-up of risk versus benefit,' Vik says later. 'Much of psychiatry is taking away a person's power when they are ill, and giving it back to them in manageable bites as they get better.' Though I'm still junior, I do not like this idea at all, but I haven't got the confidence – or knowledge – to challenge Vik with my belief that people suffering from mental illness are often completely powerless already.

I think of other areas of nursing: of intensive care, where life-support machines take over people's bodies when they are sick, gradually reducing as their organs get better. Mental-health professionals like Vik and Sue provide a kind of life-support machine for Derek's mind. Nursing, Sue tells me, is sometimes simply listening for a while, providing reassurance, keeping people safe until they can keep themselves safe. Catching the bad dreams, until a person wakes.

Derek is coming to the end of his stay, and much of Sue's work is what she calls 'therapeutic communication' and 'discharge planning' – a complex multidisciplinary affair in mental-health nursing. 'People might have been erratic and violent while ill, before admission; they may have been self-medicating with drugs and alcohol; will almost certainly have employment and money issues to sort out. So sending someone home is complex. They may not have a home any more, or it may be somewhere that is not suitable.'

Alongside a national social-housing crisis, mental illness is reaching epidemic proportions in the UK. I would imagine that all of us get mentally ill at some stage of our lives, just as we get physically ill. I've certainly felt better and worse at various times of my life, both mentally and physically. But one in four of us gets ill enough to be diagnosed with a mental-health condition. One in ten children now has a diagnosable mental illness. Suicide is on the increase, and the waiting times for people with mental illness are shameful. A government taskforce recently condemned years of under-investment in mental-health resources and found that the average maximum wait for a community mental-health-team appointment is thirty weeks. Mental-health wards are working above capacity and are breaching guidelines. Prime Minister Theresa May has promised a revolution in mental-health services and has announced 21,000 new mental-health jobs. But with the mental-health nurse's student bursary being scrapped, it is difficult to see where these nurses will come from. Janet Davies, Chief Executive and General Secretary of the Royal College of Nursing, has said, 'There is already a dangerous lack of workforce planning and accountability... Under this government, there are 5,000 fewer mental-health nurses and that goes some way to explaining why patients are being failed.'

Mental illness is devastating. After spending some time on the ward with people who are frightened and vulnerable, and sometimes desperately ill for a long time, I agree with Sue: 'I'd rather have cancer than a serious mental illness.'

But it is not just the UK that is struggling with mental health. The UN recognises mental health as a global priority. In China, where mental illness used to be thought of as political evil rather than an organic disease, there are now 100 million sufferers of mental illness. In an age when we have everything, when our living conditions are better, when our general health and education should be at a universally higher standard, we are suffering as never before.

I notice that Derek seems afraid whenever he is near Pam. He paces up and down and starts showing the body language that suggests stress: clenched jaw, eyes down, closing his body in on itself, shutting out the world. I have the chance to talk with him in the dining room. Pam – the pale, thin woman suffering with depression – is queuing up with her tray in perfect order, a huge smile on her face. The dining room is filled with staff and patients eating lunch. Food is eaten too quickly, or too slowly, and there is a high incidence of choking in mental-health settings. Sometimes patients choke deliberately, in an attempt to self-harm.

People try to hurt themselves in all kinds of inventive ways: tying ligatures around their necks; sexual self-mutilation, such as attempting to cut off a penis; burning skin or pulling out hair; swallowing razor blades, needles, pins or batteries;

drinking bleach or anti-freeze; picking at skin, cutting it. Self-harm has always existed, but there remains no clear understanding as to why, although self-harm is considered by some sufferers as a narrative, a sort of language. There is no greater expression of pain than a person who eats so little they may die. Or eats so much they may die. Obesity is self-harm. Addiction is self-harm. We hurt ourselves in different ways to express such emotional pain.

In her book *Psyche on the Skin: A History of Self-Harm*, Sarah Chaney, who works for the Royal College of Nursing, describes psychiatric narratives as being just as constructed as historical, literary or artistic narratives of self-injury. There is a distinction to be made, however, between self-harm and attempted suicide. 'Frida Kahlo committed suicide aged forty-seven,' Derek says. 'Everyone said it was a blood clot in her lung, but it was an overdose.'

It's the first time I hear him talking about suicide. Sue is sitting opposite him. 'Do you ever think of it?' she asks.

'Suicide?' He narrows his eyes. 'Doesn't everyone?'

She shakes her head. 'I don't think so, no.'

Derek is wearing a woollen hat with a Nike symbol on the front. 'When I was smoking a lot of gear. Foolish me.'

'You've stopped now, though,' she says.

'If you concentrate really hard, even while you dream that you can change the place you're dreaming. I walk backwards into this dream instead of forwards.'

I have no idea what Derek means, but we sit a while and I simply listen. He seems calm: his body is relaxed and he smiles more easily. There is no anger in his eyes and there is no fear there, either.

But Sue is frowning. 'I don't think he should go on day-release,' she tells me later. 'He needs reviewing. Psychiatry is like a blind man in a dark room, looking for a black cat that isn't really there. I think Oliver Sacks wrote that. Or a version of it. Insight can be a dangerous thing.'

I have no idea what Derek was talking about, or what Sue is talking about. Or what Oliver Sacks was talking about. But it all feels important.

I am the first to find him. Derek is lying on the floor next to his bed with blood spewing out of his arm in a grotesquely beautiful arc. The blood is redder than you could ever imagine. His eyes are open, but his skin is grey ash.

I stand for many seconds – too many seconds – unable to move my legs or close my mouth. The smell of the sea, and old chess sets, and the sound of his laughing is all replaced with nothing. For a moment or two I am with Derek, somewhere else. Hovering.

Hayley screams from outside the door. A small pair of scissors lie a foot away from Derek, near his outstretched hand. Then: rushing at the blood and the emergency buzzer, and shouting all at once and the room fills up with people far more qualified than I am to deal with such an emergency. A doctor runs in and another, and by the time the crash team from the main hospital arrives, I am kneeling on the floor, in pools of red, red blood. It looks like oil, patterned. Someone gives me a glove. 'Put pressure on it. Press as hard as you can.'

Derek's arm is so criss-crossed with red that it's difficult to see where he's managed to break through the skin and dig through flesh to find a vein – or is it an artery? The blood is exploding out in a torrent. There are cuts all up his arm, some of them deep with the flesh bursting out, others less deep but bleeding more. One cut spews blood. I press with gauze that becomes soaked in seconds. Eventually, though, my fingers press hard on the right spot and I hold firm and tight, whilst a trickle of blood still escapes. I can barely hear the shouts:

'Tourniquet!'

'Straight to theatre!'

'Crash bloods!'

I remember thinking about the colour of blood, how impossibly red it is. How different from what you'd imagine. How warm it is, almost hot. I try to estimate the amount, and only come up with far too much.

Slowly Derek begins to cough, and move his other arm. Everything slows.

'It's okay. You're going to be okay,' someone says. He turns his face to a nurse standing by the door. 'Call ahead to A&E – we'll get him over there now,' he says.

I hate blood. And here it is, covering my hand and my arm. Here is blood, the reddest, warmest blood – the very thing I wanted to avoid. And yet the lightness at the back of my head does not happen. I do not faint. I do not feel dizzy. I press so hard on Derek's forearm that my fingers are entirely numb. All I do is focus on his face, screwed up tightly and afraid, small shards of tears appearing at the corner of his eyelids like tiny fragments of glass. Derek's face is full of fear. I want to scoop him up somehow. To wrap him in a blanket and keep him safe. I want to fight some invisible power that means he is more likely to be ill, more likely to be diagnosed and more likely to be detained.

Derek looks out of the window, somewhere far away. I watch Sue put her hands on him and whisper gently into his ear, until his face is less afraid. I want to know what she is whispering and, although I can't quite hear the words, I understand something about mental-health nursing from it. Good mental-health nurses save lives. And with the biggest government cuts of all to services within the NHS, and to social care, mental-health services – and mental-health nurses – are now at breaking point. Mental-health services are a hand grenade with no pin. There aren't enough dream-catchers in the world.

3

The Origins of the World

We come spinning out of nothingness, scattering stars like dust.

Jalaluddin Rumi

Like the nurses and doctors who run towards terrorists, Florence Nightingale ran towards danger. She left her privileged upper-middle-class upbringing and the expectation that she would marry, maintain a lovely home, act as hostess and bring up children. Instead, Nightingale enrolled at the Institution of Protestant Deaconesses at Kaiserswerth in Germany, where she learned basic nursing skills, training for two weeks in July 1850 and then for a further three months in July 1851. In 1854 she travelled to Scutari in Turkey, to attend to soldiers wounded in the Crimean War, where during her first winter there 4,077 soldiers died. Ten times more soldiers died from illnesses such as typhus, typhoid, cholera and dysentery than died from battle wounds. Nightingale replaced parlour games and needlework with 'appalling horror ... steeped up to our necks in blood'. On her return to Britain, she took a keen interest in the training and development of nurses and the midwifery unit of St Thomas's Hospital – where Florence Nightingale was involved with the associated midwifery training school.

The requirements for midwives in the past now seem pretty offensive. John Maubray wrote in *The Female Physician* of 1724: 'She ought not to be too fat or gross, but especially not to have thick or fleshy hands and arms, or large-bon'd wrists...'

Along with the treatment of midwives, the treatment and care of mothers has changed beyond recognition in both the US and the UK since then. Fertility in the over-forty age group has trebled since the 1980s, and there are now more women giving birth in their forties than in their teens. Even without fertility, it is increasingly possible to conceive. More American women now receive medical help (IVF) to have their babies than ever before, according to a report from the Society for Assisted Reproductive Technology. The way in which women give birth is also changing. In 2014 guidance from NICE was updated to focus on enabling women greater freedom to choose where they give birth; there is evidence that midwife-led units are safer than hospital, for women who are expected to have a straightforward, low-risk birth. Community and home births are slowly increasing and are set to rise over the coming years. Conversely Caesarean sections are also rising and now account for around one in four births in the UK.

Practices before and after birth vary wildly throughout the world. The association of childbirth with lying-in, or confinement, is centuries old, and although it is now outdated in the West, it is still widely practised around the world. In China women do nothing for a period of thirty days, being confined inside, prior to their due date. And yet in America, the only industrialised nation not to mandate paid maternity leave, and where forty-three million American workers have no paid sick leave, a quarter of new mothers return to work less than two weeks after giving birth. What happens to the secure attachment of babies towards their mother? Do a quarter of American babies develop an attachment disorder? In Europe, too, there are wide differences in hospital practice. In France, women stay for a minimum of three days in hospital after giving birth. In the UK, women can be discharged within a few hours.

'Childbirth is a natural process, not an illness,' Frances, the midwife whom I am shadowing, tells me. Student mental-health nurses do not have to spend time in midwifery but my first-year group is offered a placement on the labour wards and I jump at the chance. Frances's voice is brisk, matching the way she marches around the room, tidying as she goes, putting blood- and fluid-soiled incontinence pads into yellow clinical waste bins, washing her hands, straightening the sheets. Frances shows me around, and I follow her as she walks through the antenatal ward, 'where we care for women who are more than twenty weeks pregnant who are unwell'; the day assessment unit, for 'problems in pregnancy. We can do ultrasounds, bloods – that kind of thing.' We pass a room where a woman is hooked up to a CTG (cardiotocography) machine that measure foetal heartbeats and uterine contractions, and where the terror of stillbirth hangs in the air. We pass women who are suffering from hyperemesis gravida – extreme morning sickness – and need drips to replenish their fluid, after continual vomiting day and night. There are women with gestational diabetes, growing enormous babies. Some women are simply anxious and have nothing physically wrong with them, but have lost a baby (or five) previously, and their fear of it happening again is acute and achingly painful. There are women who have other conditions during their pregnancy, such as heart complaints, asthma or immune-system disorders, and who have to take medication that is unlicensed during pregnancy, weighing up the risks and benefits.

Frances tells me how the evidence shows that women with uncomplicated pregnancies who are cared for on the mid-wifery-led unit are more likely to have a normal birth, and to require less pain relief. A woman is screaming from one of the side-rooms.

We walk past the induction-of-labour rooms to the hand-over office, where I get a flash of the huge whiteboard that lists the women: room number, gestation, parity (how many babies they've had), summary of condition, progress, analgesia and the name of the midwife assigned to her. There is a pool room to my right, then seven labour rooms and, at the end, a multiple-birth room. In the centre of the pool room is a giant paddling pool, and a kind of swing hanging above it that the women can use to pull themselves around. The men can get in, too, Frances says, though it can get messy. 'A bit like *Jaws*.'

There's a small mesh net hidden at the back of the pool, which the midwife uses to fish out shit or vomit; and there are speakers to play music. I overhear the midwives talking about first-time mothers as they eat large slabs of stale birthday cake left by the night staff. 'They arrive at the labour ward one centimetre dilated with a laminated birth plan requesting relaxing music, aromatherapy oils and refusing all pain relief until things really get going. Then they scream for everything we have in the meds cupboards. The ones with a doula are the worst.'

But Frances is a fan of doulas – experienced women who have received some training in births. 'It makes sense to me that doulas would be part of a birth plan.' Much like the traditional birth attendants that pre-dated midwives prior to the eighteenth century, a doula is a birth companion or post-birth supporter: a champion of the woman in labour. The research I've read suggests that women who have the support of a doula – who stays with them continually throughout their labour – have shorter delivery times, fewer Caesarean sections, and their babies spend less time in neonatal intensive care.

I learn that there are many different types of midwives, even within the same speciality. The midwives are split between medicalised and traditional: those who are interested in such things as advanced neonatal life support, and those who are totally averse to medical intervention unless absolutely necessary. This conflict within midwifery started outside it. From the eighteenth century onwards, conflict arose between surgeons and midwives, as medical men began to assert that their modern scientific techniques were better for mothers and infants than the folk medicine practised by midwives.

Midwives are no longer involved with traditional folk medicine in the UK, but rather in what could be considered a nod to it. But in other countries – Nigeria, for example – it is perfectly usual to find traditional birth attendants in rural areas. The other extreme is the United States, where obstetricians (doctors) run the show, with midwife-nurses on hand to help. American women are, however, increasingly choosing midwife-nurses over obstetricians to deliver their babies. There are many ways to be both a midwife and a nurse, and the spectrum between medicalised and traditional roles depends on the individual, as opposed to the speciality. For instance, while Florence Nightingale ran the general hospital at Scutari, Mary Seacole set up a boarding house and shop, where she sold remedies for walk-ins. What was in the remedies she did not specify. Maybe she understood that it did not matter.

Frances stands in the middle of the traditional-versus-modern way of practising. She is an experienced midwife who was a scientist in what she calls 'a previous life'. She retrained after having her own children, and now works on a combination of consultant-led and midwife-led wards, as she is on today. 'I've been doing this job for years now, and have delivered hundreds of babies,' she tells me. 'Maybe thousands. And it never gets old.'

She is wearing dark-blue scrubs and black clogs, which mean that even when she is walking quickly she appears relaxed. She has ironed a fold in the short sleeves of her top, sharp and perfect. Her face is perfectly made-up and she does not have a hair out of place.

I am already a sweaty mess just following Frances around, and my hair is out of control. The labour ward is hot and humid. I can feel my own hurriedly applied make-up sliding off my face. We are caring for Scarlett, a young woman in the early stages of labour.

'Young mum,' says Frances. 'First baby. You can't predict how it will go. Some of my women look fragile enough that they will break, and they pop a baby out like shelling a pea. Others look as tough as nails, and end up going down a pathway of medicalisation: drugs, epidural, forceps, C-section. You can't tell.'

Scarlett is sitting up when we go in. I hover by the door.

'Come in,' Frances ushers me in, waving her hand. 'This is Christie, she's a student with me today. She's here to observe, if that's okay with you.'

Scarlett nods. 'I don't care if the army observes,' she says. 'I just want it out.' She laughs. She is wearing a once-white bra that has been washed greyish. She has a tattoo on her shoulder that says 'Rocket'. Is Rocket the father? Her breasts are enormous and covered in blue-green veins. Her stomach is impossibly big and shining. She looks young, too young to have a baby. I remember my friend who was pregnant at twelve and had a baby at thirteen; she came to my house for tea and a play one day after school, armed with a baby. I remember my dad's face. 'What the bleeding hell?'

Scarlett is single – 'he didn't stick around, but thank God for small mercies' – and does not have a doula, although she has her mum with her, who is clutching her hand. Scarlett laughs and looks at me. 'Seriously, I don't care. I just want this baby out of me.' She has red hair and freckles.

'More likely to tear. Thin skin,' Frances later tells me. 'And she's young. Horrendous stretch marks, but the muscles recover really well.'

The room is bathed in sunlight. It is too hot, actually, and the windows do not open. Frances has found a broken fan that is stuck facing in one direction, but still blows out air at number three. She angles it towards Scarlett's face. Despite the fan, there are drops of sweat patterning her skin. Her mum reaches over with a grey flannel and dabs Scarlett's forehead. 'There, that's nice and cool. I have glucose tablets, too, Scar, that you can have. Well prepared.'

Scarlett's mum is wearing a T-shirt that says 'Mexico' across her chest, with a picture of a palm tree. She notices me looking at it. 'We went four years ago. Best holiday ever. The food! Ate so many cheese tacos I thought I'd turn into one.'

Scarlett rolls her eyes, then pushes the flannel away. 'I'm going to puke,' she says.

Frances pushes past me and arrives just in time with a small cardboard sick-bowl underneath Scarlett's chin. 'Don't worry, happens all the time. You won't be sick when the baby is out.' Had she been carrying a sick-bowl with her, just in case, all along? I hadn't noticed one.

A giant bouncy beach ball, like a space hopper without the handles, rolls back and forth towards Scarlett's bed. I discover later that it is a birthing ball, which women sit on to promote good posture in labour. There is an outfit laid out on the bassinet next to the window: a Winnie-the-Pooh Babygro, hat and booties in yellow. Evidence of a McDonald's takeaway lines the windowsill: a large cardboard cup, burger packets, chip wrappers. There's a small bathroom with a large bin next to the toilet and a sign: 'Don't throw away the sanitary pads. I need to see the clots and check everything is all okay after the birth. Just pop them on top of the bin.'

When the midwife tells Scarlett it's time to see how she's progressing and opens Scarlett's legs, I almost fall over. Botticelli's *The Birth of Venus*, painted in the 1480s and depicting the goddess Venus emerging from a seashell on the shore, represents the metaphor – used since classical antiquity – of a seashell as a woman's vulva. I love that painting.

Scarlett's vulva is nothing like a seashell.

The shock of seeing the swollen, torn skin, the transparent stretching of a balloon about to pop, sends me back to my childhood bedroom, and I'm a skinny girl again, holding a seashell to my ear. I can almost feel the cold of it. I search for my dad's words: 'If you listen hard you can hear nothing and everything, all at the same time,' but all I hear is screaming.

This is the first time I watch a baby being born. From the beginning of Scarlett's pushing, I have been crying and shocked, convinced something has gone wrong. I was warned that the umbilical cord is blue, and the baby's head will be the shape of an ice-cream cone. But the violence of the pushing shocks me.

I am a new and completely novice nurse, and although I am beginning to know the theory, I haven't yet experienced anything outside the classroom. Patricia Benner, a nursing theorist, describes my stage of development as 'knowing that', but not yet 'knowing how'. But in this room, seeing Scarlett somewhere on the edge of life and her baby creeping towards it, I feel as if I know nothing at all.

I am crying and crying. Frances glances at me and frowns, but I can't stop. After all the screaming, Scarlett goes very quiet. Then she makes a low groaning that does not sound human. In past centuries, a birth was sometimes called a 'groaning' or a 'crying out'. Visiting guests, friends and family celebrating a child's birth were even offered 'groaning beer' and 'groaning cake'. I know this. Yet still I am not prepared for the sound. I count the beads of sweat appearing on Scarlett's face, covering her freckles. I try not to think about her skin. The thinness of it. The tearing.

'I want an epidural,' she screams. 'I can't do it. I can't push any more.'

Frances is calm at first. 'Let's give it another contraction. Then I'll organise it. Okay?'

The groaning gets louder, more foreign and further away from Scarlett's natural voice, as if coming from another place. It sounds like a noise belonging to the earth, from long ago and far away. Scarlett is pushing and panting and writhing around on the bed as if she's on fire. That can't be normal. And Frances has half a hand inside her, gloves covered in slime, her eyes looking almost through Scarlett's stomach.

'I'm dying,' Scarlett shouts.

Scarlett's mum starts crying, too, and doesn't stop, until the M of the word 'Mexico' is soaked a different colour from the other letters.

Frances pulls her hands away and opens a sterile white delivery pack at the base of the bed. Her voice changes and becomes hard. 'You are not dying. You need to push harder. You can do it. Well done, you're doing so well.'

Scarlett stops screaming and thrashing around.

The baby is born with a caul over its head – a kind of papery bag, the amniotic membrane covering the foetus, which usually remains inside the mother. Frances loops it off the baby's head as simply as if taking off a hat.

'Right. Good girl. Now I want you to pant, then push gently when I tell you.'

The baby's head is out, and the rest comes in a rush of blood and shit and sticky white stuff. There is gunky fluid everywhere, and the walls are alive with Scarlett's screaming. Frances rubs the back of the baby as if towel-drying hair, then plonks it on Scarlett's chest.

'It's a girl,' she says.

Scarlett sobs. 'A girl.' Her body convulses and shakes. 'A girl!'

'Don't worry about this.' Frances gestures to the caul. 'Some say it's a sign that the baby will be destined for greatness.' And she expresses happy surprise as if it's her first time.

I watch Scarlett's face as she gazes at her newborn and at her mother, and the look that passes between them makes me cry even more. The sound of Scarlett's daughter crying is one of the nicest noises I've ever heard, a strange and beautiful music.

Frances is still busy. After delivering the placenta, and cutting the cord, she has a stitching kit out, ready to fix Scarlett's too-thin skin. 'Very bad tears can even leave a woman incontinent, and are more common than you'd think.' Research from the *British Journal of Gynaecology* found that 85 per cent of women experience some form of tear during their first vaginal birth.

Luckily, Scarlett – despite her thin skin – does not fall into the 'severe' category of trauma: what obstetricians refer to as 'obstetric anal sphincter injury' (because the tissue has torn all the way to the anus and has caused nerve as well as muscle damage). She does not need to go to theatre to be operated on, in order to hopefully repair the damage. She still has a small tear, but it is 'level two', meaning that Frances can stitch it up herself. But before she does so, she takes a moment to kneel down next to Scarlett and admire the baby. 'She's perfect,' she says. She strokes the baby's cheek, then reaches out and strokes Scarlett's cheek. 'Lucky you, and lucky her. Well done, Mum.'

I have to leave the room. I lean on the wall outside, next to the red fire extinguisher and the cork board full of baby photos. I am in pieces. Childbirth is a bloody business. My head feels light and my eyes dizzy. But it is not the gore that I think of. The air is different. The world is different. My student nurse's dress collar is wet with tears, but they continue to fall. I am in total amazement at women, at midwives, at humanity.

Later, in the dirty utility room, Frances shows me how to check the placenta. She lays it in a plastic tray. It's bigger than I imagine. 'Look for clear bubbles on the outside,' she says. 'Can be a sign of gestational diabetes, or congenital hearts.' She talks as she examines the organ. It looks like liver that you'd find at any butcher's, though slightly lighter: a deep maroon, the colour of Pinot Noir. 'This around the cord is Wharton's jelly – contained also in the eyeball.'

I look at the gelatinous substance and try not to gag. 'It looks like the inside of a pork pie,' I say.

'Quite,' she replies, not smiling.

'It was so animalistic,' I say to Frances. 'She groaned like an animal. I don't know how to describe it, but otherworldly, non-human. Like a cow!'

Frances glances up at me, then flicks her eyes back to the placenta. 'Normal.'

Human labour is quite different from labour in other species. There are plenty of studies which show that a complex biochemical dialogue occurs between the mother and foetus and the placenta. The human placenta lacks the enzyme CYP17, which stimulates labour in animals. Labour in humans is more of a language – a language between mother and baby, translated by the placenta, like the one Frances is holding in front of her. The secret language of women.

'Giving birth is the most natural, human thing of all,' she says. 'There is no greater expression of humanity.'

She has a way of explaining things so that I understand, in a way that I don't understand. 'Birth holds the hand of death,' she tells me. 'We begin and we end at the same time.'

It is 1998 and I am finally a qualified nurse. I decided not to stay in mental-health nursing, finding the sadness too sad, and swapped specialities to children's nursing. I love that although children get very ill very quickly they recover even faster, most of the time. I move into a flat in south-east London with my three best friends, who are all student midwives. I reminisce, tell them my one experience of midwifery thus far: 'Scarlett was so brave. And young. It was ordinary; it was extraordinary!' My friends smile at each other with their eyes. They are already halfway through their required forty deliveries to train to be midwives. They buy Tarot cards – 'midwives used all to be witches' – and tell me my future in the evenings, with church candles lighting up the Robbie Williams posters that are Blu-tacked to the Artexed living-room wall, and a shelf full of corks with the occasion written on them in biro: 'Tuesday evening, shit day', 'Friday pre-clubbing', 'Nic's birthday – vodka-jelly night'.

'You will meet a dark, handsome stranger,' my friends say. 'And travel the world. You will live until you are a hundred years old.' Or one evening, after I made too much noise the night before, when my flatmate was on an early shift: 'I see some tragedy. You will face uncertainty, and there are knives in your back.'

They dread the full-moon shifts. There is no scientific evidence that more babies are born during full moons, but I've lived with three midwives: science must be wrong. The morning after a full-moon shift they are always late, stressed and more tired: 'Haven't sat down all night! Completely full, and backed up. It's no wonder we all try and roster ourselves on crescent-moon weekends.'

They accumulate a billion more stories, but listen graciously as I try and describe to them the feeling of watching such a miracle during my early training, which is their daily bread and butter. 'It's hard to put into words what you do. I mean, you are somewhere at the centre of why we are – the state of all life.' I listen, too, after they've had a bad day, and swear never to moan about a bad day at the office.

'The baby was long dead. She said it had stopped moving days ago and she was too scared to tell anyone. She was in labour for ten hours. We tried to speed things up, but she refused all medication. Said she wanted to give birth to her son. She pushed for over an hour.'

'The shoulder was stuck: shoulder dystocia. McRoberts manoeuvre didn't work. The doctor had to break the baby's collarbone inside the mother. The baby shot across the room like a football.'

'The baby was born with an encephalocele – literally a brain outside its head. The mum held him, but the dad left. He couldn't look at the baby. To be honest, I found it hard to look.'

To cope, we have parties all the time. We live in a sprawling Victorian house in a dodgy bit of the city that is split into flats, with another group of student midwives upstairs, and us in the middle. The downstairs flat is empty and we are concerned: who will put up with our noise? We regularly have friends with giant speakers and all-night bedroom DJ sets blasting through the old building. When we see the two young, good-looking men walking up the road with the estate agent, we are drinking cocktails and are all still wearing nightwear. It is noon (we have finished five night shifts). My midwife friend leans out of the window.

'Hi! You looking at the downstairs flat?'

Before getting to the gate, one of the men turns to the estate agent. 'We'll take it.'

Like all nurses, midwives and doctors, we keep odd hours. Tuesdays are sometimes Saturdays, and we are just as likely to have a big night on a Monday morning as most people would on a Saturday night. On consecutive days off, we drink cheap wine and hooch. We climb out of the toilet window and sit on the roof of a condemned building, smoking; or, once, finishing a canister of nitrous oxide that is left over from a home birth. Although nitrous oxide is commonplace in the UK, in America it is far less frequently prescribed. Judith Rooks, a certified US nurse-midwife, makes the point that 'No one makes a lot of money when a woman uses nitrous oxide.'

It remains a safe and helpful analgesia for women in labour in the NHS, but is also used as oxidiser in rocket propellants. We are not the first people to abuse it for pleasure: from 1799 the British upper classes would have laughing-gas parties. We are soon screaming with laughter, watching the London sunset, the sky streaked with red.

But the parties do not last. And my friends are right about tragedy after all, with their Tarot cards and their talk of witch-craft. Life changes for all of us within a period of six months. One of us loses his mum to cancer; another has a friend die in a flash-flood accident in Arizona; and one of my best friends, Callum, whom I grew up with, dies by suicide.

When Callum hangs himself on New Year's Eve, my entire world is streaked with red. I think about depression. About suicide. About freedom. About Derek. I revisit the small schoolroom where fifteen-year-old Callum and I were separated from our classmates, deemed clever and encour-aged to self-study. We ignored our books and instead had conversations about Camus; and I remember the gold-tipped Russian cigarettes we smoked, which we completely believed made us appear intellectual. I remember my friend's hair, and Scarlett's; how he was red-haired and thin-skinned, too, tearing too easily. But I can't make sense of any of it.

In another life – along with my many other career aspirations at school – I'd have been a sonographer. But I don't study heart scans, as a nurse. I watch the scans happening on the computer screens, as a writer. The sensory experience of the sound of hearts, the beautiful colours of blue and red unoxygenated and oxygenated blood. The patterns we all have inside us are the most beautiful landscape you can imagine. The movement of our blood flow – we dance inside. I carry with me the sound of the whoosh of the heart scan, as some people carry the sound of a drumbeat from a favourite song. I remember beats. The smaller the baby, the faster and louder the whoosh. Babies gallop, racing to live. A scan of a baby's heart reminds me that survival is instinctive, at birth perhaps more than ever – that will of a newborn, of a species, of survival. We run towards life.

All heart scans are amazing, but some are terrifying. Some hearts beat differently, dangerously. There is a heart rhythm which occurs more commonly – and usually mainly – in children, called 'supraventricular tachycardia' (SVT), whereby the will to survive flicks into a dangerous speed, and the baby's or child's heart beats fast enough that it cannot empty enough blood around the body. But when looking after a baby with SVT, I'm reminded of where we began. The treatment involves dipping the babies face-first into iced water or, failing that, covering their faces with ice. Human babies, along with dolphins, otters and some seabirds (including penguins), have a diver's reflex until they're six months old. It is the kind of reflex that overrides other reflexes, allowing a baby to stay underwater for longer than usual without drowning. Our connection to nature, our will to survive.

If the dive reflex doesn't work, the doctors are ready with a drug called adenosine that stuns the heart; they watch the monitor as the heart trace flattens for a few of the longest seconds ever, before a normal QRS complex – the heart waves that show regular ventricular electrical activity – is present. But cold water has fewer side-effects. Adenosine is given rapidly into a vein, followed by a large water syringe, to push the drug in more quickly. Adenosine does not live in the plasma for long: it is metabolised fast by the kidneys and liver, so it needs to be given quickly to take full effect. It is described as leaving a patient with a sense of impending doom. A more accurate explanation is that the patient will feel as if they have died for a few seconds, while their heart stops. They will be flatline – asystolic – while the heart is stunned, then electrical activity will, hopefully, recommence in a normal way. It is a terrifying pause.

'Think of it like an orchestra,' a doctor tells me. 'The flutes are playing one thing, the cellos another, and nobody is listening to anyone. The music sounds terrible. Interventions like adenosine or synchronised cardioversion are the conductor raising the baton. There are a few seconds of silence, before everybody begins to play again, in time and in tune.'

I think of that pause between life and death. A few seconds of silence.

Congenital heart disease occurs in about eight of every 1,000 normal pregnancies. Heart disease is something we associate with poor lifestyle choices, and heart attacks are familiar in older people who eat the wrong food, drink the wrong drinks, smoke or are sedentary. Worryingly, the NHS is seeing increasing numbers of young people with this type of heart disease, along with rising numbers of obesity in younger children – even primary-school children. But a congenital heart disorder means that something has gone wrong genetically during pregnancy, whereby the child's heart has developed a hole or a structural abnormality. A foetal cardiologist once said to me that it wasn't a wonder why so many children are born with abnormalities, but more of a wonder why some children are not.

Three out of eight of these children will not live. They will live for hours or days or weeks, but adulthood will probably not be a possibility. These are the lost children. The families who give birth to a perfect-looking baby, knowing that inside them is a diseased heart that will not last them long enough. A faulty clock that will stop. Their entire lives simply a few seconds of silence.

I am by now working on a Paediatric Intensive-Care Unit, where there are a number of general patients, but also a section on a different floor specifically for cardiac patients. The ward has a four-bedded area around the corner from the theatres. There are no windows, and the lighting is a strange kind of artificial neon. But children do not stay here long. It's a halfway gap between the operation and the cardiac ward, between life and death. The beds are all in a row, with nothing separating them. Alongside the back wall are drawers and drawers of equipment: syringes, saline flushes, gauze and Tegaderm dressings, miniature pairs of scissors, rolls of Elastoplast, long white ribbon tapes for securing tubes. The children and babies are mostly here post-cardiac surgery, wheeled straight from theatre by the surgeon and anaesthetist, and near enough to the operating rooms to go back, if necessary.

Each patient has various accessories: thin wires attached to boxes that look like portable speakers, which can pace a child if their heart flicks into a different rhythm: take over the electrics. They usually have thick tubes the size of large earthworms coming from their sides, attached to large, rectangular drainage boxes on the floor underneath the beds, where excess blood can drain out. The nurses check regularly that these are swinging and bubbling, in order to know that they are working and are not blocked. Occasionally the patient dumps a load of blood, and the fullness of the drains tells the nurse that they are bleeding to death and need to get back to theatre, and the surgeons, before it's too late.

I look after a baby with stiff lungs (pulmonary hypertension), as the heart has been pumping too hard, and for too long, with a valve that doesn't work and a hole in the centre. She will not self-oxygenate and needs to go onto nitric oxide in order to live. Nitric oxide is not to be confused with the nitrous oxide that my midwife friends and I were inhaling. Nitric oxide, which is used regularly in neonatal, child and adult Intensive-Care Units in the high-oxygen-rich environment of the ventilation circuit, has the dangerous potential to convert to cytotoxic nitrogen oxide – the same gas that was produced by nuclear tests and was responsible for the reddish colour in mushroom clouds. Another gas used in hospitals, heliox, runs out so quickly that an entire day is spent rushing around the hospital with empty cylinders. Heliox (helium and oxygen) has the side-effect of changing the baby's voice when she is extubated – when the breathing tube is removed. Her voice is the same, but as heliox is lighter, it makes the sound travel faster, so it sounds higher. Words travel faster on lighter air.

'Heliox is the stuff of helium balloons,' I tell the baby, talking to her over the whoosh of her oxygen mask. 'And the reason we know that dolphins don't actually whistle. They tested dolphins whistling in air and heliox, and the heliox helped to prove it.' The baby looks up at me, her eyes wide. I laugh, lift her onto my lap and make up a story about a dolphin. But not every day is for stories and cuddles.

When I started nursing, I imagined nothing more upsetting than caring for sick babies. But I look after a child who, for no apparent reason, has cardiomyopathy – an enlarged heart. A teenager. I watch her face, the tiny prongs of oxygen in her nose. She looks at the X-ray the doctor holds up, showing the size of her heart taking up too much space. She will not live. 'I have too much heart?' she asks.

All childbirth is extreme. The edge of our experience, as human beings. Much later, the delivery of my own daughter teaches me that. I am lying with my legs in stirrups, with people coming in and out of the room, shaking hands with the dad, who is a doctor and knows everyone. They greet my vagina (which I'm fairly certain looks nothing like a shell), but I am beyond caring. I feel as if I am being run over by a truck, slowly. I have a medicalised birth, and a room full of alarms, doctors, machines. My daughter, who is stuck, is pulled out of me with instruments. A haemorrhage. But still, it is considered normal.

Even Scarlett's labour – a completely normal birth – felt totally otherworldly. Watching a child being born is one thing, and all childbirth is unbelievable. But watching a child being born when the parents know the baby has a serious and potentially life-limiting illness is quite a different experience. A not-normal delivery.

Baby Murphy might not be going home. Claire Murphy is pressing her chin down onto her chest and I can hear the sound of her teeth grinding together. Her midwife, Preeti, is a small woman, wearing dark-purple scrubs and an apron. There are lots of people in the room: a paediatrician, a neonatologist (newborns' doctor), and another midwife I don't recognise hovers next to a resuscitaire, a kind of incubator with an overhead heater and dials, allowing oxygen and air to be pumped through a small bag to help the baby breathe, if necessary. Claire's husband, Richard, stands by her side, stroking her hair and cheek. He looks as if he's about to fall over. His other hand is clutching the back of a plastic chair, his shoulders moving with each of his breaths. The midwife by the resuscitaire is talking to the doctors about settings. But despite all the people in the room, the only ones are really Claire and her midwife.

'Listen to my voice,' says Preeti. 'You are going to do this. We will do it together. I can see your baby's head. Lots of hair already.' She is at the bottom of the bed looking up, gloves on, a delivery pack open, towels ready – one to wipe the gunk, then one to warm the baby.

Claire is wearing a T-shirt, nothing on her bottom half, but is covered with a sheet and she has socks on, the fluffy kind that you might see during winter, purple-and-pink-striped. She looks round, her head moving from side to side. She does not cry in pain. Nor does she push. There is a machine next to her that is measuring the baby's heartbeat in waves and beeps, and the alarm keeps sounding.

'Don't worry about that,' Preeti says. 'Only my voice. On the next contraction I want you to push a bit. Not hard-hard – the baby is nearly out. But a bit.'

The doctors look at each other. 'Shall we get Claudette?'

I understand that Claudette is the senior obstetrician. The doctor who can perform C-sections, or pull the baby out with a ventouse (a kind of suction cup) or forceps.

Preeti looks up and changes the tone in her voice. 'We do not need help here. Claire is birthing her baby without help.'

Midwifery is a strange art. It is not about the technical aspects of the equipment that can facilitate a birth, but much more about judgement. Preeti tells me, 'An experienced midwife can know everything about a woman: whether she will be pushing the baby out or not, whether she will cope without an epidural, and when to answer her question about getting one. Because we know.' This is entirely different to what Frances told me years ago. Like nursing, midwifery has many accents.

But Claire does not look as if she is pushing hard enough. Preeti half-stands and looks straight at her. 'If you do not push now, we will have to get help. I know we discussed that, and it's not what you want. So you need to do what you wanted. You can do this.'

Claire takes a breath. She is crying. 'I don't want it to end,' she says. 'I can't. What if?'

She looks up at Richard. He is crying now, too. The room is quiet. Even the alarms on the machine are quiet. Finally Claire pushes her head towards her chest, the crunching of teeth, then a scream.

We are in side-room ten, much like Scarlett's. There is a bathroom to the side, a few easy-to-wipe-down chairs underneath a high-up slit window, and the room is too hot. There's a pull-out tray table that you can find on all hospital wards, a wood colour on top with legs that are designed to fit under the bed. Balanced on it are a large jug of water and a few cups. I stand at the bottom of the bed, near enough that if the baby needs resuscitating I'll be on hand, with air. I don't think about the seriousness of the situation. I am still a novice. But the air canister feels a lot heavier than it should. My arm is numb. I know little about the family, or the baby who will be arriving imminently. But I do know the baby has a condition called hypoplastic left heart syndrome, whereby the left pumping chamber and the aorta are much too small, and the heart is unable to pump enough blood around the body.

The nature of a baby with hypoplastic left heart syndrome (a 'hypoplast', as we call them) means that oxygen – the life-giving, lifesaving drug that we routinely use during medical emergencies – can kill. There is a tiny duct that is helping to keep the baby alive, their foetal underwater circulation. Usually this closes a few days after birth, but Baby Murphy's duct needs to stay open. Oxygen can speed up the closure of this hole. If these babies cry, they let in too much oxygen. Much of a nurse's job caring for a pre-stage-one Norwood procedure – the first of three major re-plumbing operations to treat hypoplastic left heart syndrome – is to make sure these babies don't cry: so much resting on such a simple thing. If Baby Murphy needs help breathing when he is born, my task is to hand over the canister of air instead.

Claire is surrounded by people. Her dark hair is fanned out over her pillow and her T-shirt is scrunched up around her middle. I focus on her fluffy pink-and-purple-striped socks. She is looking at Richard, and I watch the glance that passes between them. Fear. He stays at the top end of things and looks at his wife's face. Claire now pushes and screams and pushes.

'Listen to my voice,' Preeti says.

The neonatologist, the other midwife and the paediatrician all stand back near the equipment. I stand as close to the door as possible. I am here to make sure nobody gives oxygen. An oxygen-gatekeeper. It is a nothing job – a task that anyone can do. But I hold my breath, wishing the baby to be born okay.

Claire's face changes colour. She pants. I watch Baby Murphy come out in a rush, a flurry, an instant. Preeti has unhooked the cord, which was around the baby's neck, and reaches up to place the baby on Claire's stomach, which is already deflating like an old balloon.

'You have a son,' she says.

He cries, a tiny bit. The sound of a baby's first cry is a wonderful thing, but this time I will it to be brief. Baby Murphy cries a fraction, then stops. I exhale.

Preeti holds her hands backwards to prevent the doctors coming closer. Everyone is anxious. We all look at the baby and wait. The other midwife gets a warm towel and hands it to Preeti. The doctors edge closer still. Preeti looks back at them. 'A few seconds more,' she says.

Richard sobs. He lets go of the chair and holds Claire's face in his hands. He kisses Claire like I've never seen anyone kiss. 'A son,' he whispers. He looks at the baby. 'I don't think I can cut the cord. Can you do it?'

Claire looks down at the baby. 'Can we leave it?' She looks at Preeti. 'For just a moment longer?'

Preeti's voice is calm and clear. 'Take as long as you need.'

I care for Baby Murphy following the first of three big operations. It is known as a stage-one Norwood procedure, which makes it sound almost minor. It is a huge surgery, that involves, among other things, cutting major arteries and inserting a connection called a shunt to divert blood flow.

He is still nameless. As with many babies having cardiac surgery, his tiny chest is not yet big enough to allow for the swelling of his heart, so the surgeons have to leave his chest completely open, his walnut-sized heart frantically beating in front of me, covered by a thin piece of gauze. I remember an infestation on the ward with fruit flies. Open hearts and fruit flies. They hover around the air like dust particles. We do not know where they are coming from. The ward is stripped clean and everything is removed: the carpets, the furnishings. Until we realise that the flies are coming from the staffroom where we make coffee. 'Only go into the coffee room to make coffee from the machine,' we are told by managers. But eventually they find the nest: inside the coffee machine. We stop drinking coffee, for a while.

After much discussion, Baby Murphy's six-year-old sister, Siobhan, comes to see him in the intensive-care ward.

He is hooked up to so many machines, with swollen eyes, pacing wires sticking out of him, chest drains and lines going into him. Everyone is worried about how Siobhan will react, but is more worried about her reaction to not seeing him.

Siobhan is fearless; touches his head feather-soft, smiles a wide smile. 'My brother looks like a robot,' she says, looking at all the machinery and equipment.

And Robert Murphy gets his name.

I learn rapidly in this first intensive-care job. 'It's like a baptism of fire,' a senior nurse tells me. 'Other units are better-staffed, so junior nurses here end up caring for much sicker and more complex cases, and we often don't have a runner.' A runner is a spare nurse who can cover breaks, fetch equipment, check drugs. It is considered a luxury, but in an area such as intensive care it should be a necessity. I am in my early twenties and, with limited knowledge and understanding, caring for tiny babies who have life-threatening cardiac conditions and require high-risk surgery. But it is not the patients I learn the most from. My own 'birth' as a nurse comes from a sudden truth that, in the same way a mother and her baby are never far apart, no matter the distance, a nurse and a patient are linked for ever. And sometimes the blood through an umbilical cord flows backwards. I was not born a nurse, but was made into one by other births. Both joy and tragedy build a nurse. And we cannot predict what will happen. Baby Robert Murphy survives and thrives, despite our worst fears.

But there is another baby. A baby who is perfectly healthy on the scans. One of our own. My colleague, Stuart – a wonderful, caring nurse, who has looked after thousands of babies and children – has a beautiful, perfect baby boy who suddenly becomes seriously unwell and needs admitting to our unit: the very place where Stuart works. I don't look after his baby. He has all of the most experienced and most brilliant nurses in his cubicle, rushing in and out, and a team of the best doctors alongside them. They are the best team I've ever worked with, internationally recognised. They have years and years of clinical experience, have seen it all, and then some. Most nursing theorists agree that this reflection on clinical experience is what helps nurses create meaning from their own experiences. It is a multitude of experiences that make an expert nurse, but the ability to think deeply about them, and to search for meaning, is what a good nurse is often born with.

The team of nurses and doctors that I work with have both the expertise and the self-reflection. It is a privilege to learn from them, work alongside them and know them. They are the safest of hands. But still the nurse in charge, Katerina, comes out of the cubicle mid-morning, her face grey, her eyes red, defeated. The nurses, all in a row at the end of our patients' beds, look at her in unison. There is a terrifying pause, then a few seconds of silence, before she slowly shakes her head. Sometimes, even as a novice, I understand that there simply is no meaning.

4

At First the Infant

Nothing in life is to be feared; it is only to be understood.

Marie Curie

I have studied theories of nursing in a dry, academic language that is difficult to understand. I've tried to visualise the philosophy of nursing on the wards with the actual patients, but as soon as I am there, the philosophers and nursing theorists make even less sense. I've read Florence Nightingale's Environmental Theory, where she argued that the environment is crucial to a patient's recovery. She stated that 'the greater part of nursing consists in preserving cleanliness'. I try and remember that, although it is little comfort when nursing seems to be nothing but clearing up body fluids: I spend my time wiping blood off a wall; soaking off rock-solid dried poo from a baby's back and neck; and scrubbing instruments and equipment in soapy water with Milton disinfectant tablets thrown in, which is strong enough to make my eyes stream.

Another day, nursing is simply paperwork: I write care plan after care plan, document observations and numbers, and sign a thousand signatures to confirm I've checked the right drug, right patient, right time. Another nursing day is checking: stock levels, expiry dates, equipment set up correctly, enough stationery in the stationery cupboard. Even on the varied days, when nursing ranges from running to collect a child from theatre, to dealing with medical emergencies on the ward, and comforting a relative, giving or explaining bad news, the theories bear little relation to what I'm actually doing.

Nursing expert Hildegard Peplau first developed the Interpersonal Theory in the 1960s, and identified nursing as a healing art: the nurse and patient work together, so that both become mature and knowledgeable in the process. I do not feel mature, however. Most days I feel overwhelmed, and some days completely out of my depth. On other days I feel disgusted, and occasionally simply bored and tired. Virginia Henderson, a nurse and researcher, has been described as the most influential nurse of the twentieth century. I've read her Need Theory and have tried to understand her famous definition of nursing:

> The unique function of the nurse is to assist the individual, sick or well, in the performance of those activities contributing to health or its recovery (or to peaceful death) that he would perform unaided if he had the necessary strength, will or knowledge.

> Nursing people means doing for them what they would normally do, when they have no will to do it, until they have will to do it.

I go shopping for my neighbour, who feels under the weather. I cook for a friend who has a new baby. I go to the post office for my nan, and to the bookies for my dad. But it doesn't feel like nursing. And then I read a grand nursing theory developed between 1959 and 2001 by Dorothea Orem, another nursing theorist, who says that people should be self-reliant and responsible for their own care. My head is full of conflicting arguments about what nursing actually is.

I absorb textbooks about childhood development, health and disease. I learn much about the philosophy of attachment, and study the work on child development by psychologist and psychiatrist John Bowlby, and I become fascinated with the ethics of Harry Harlow's work on attachment. In one of his studies, baby monkeys were left alone in darkness for up to one year from birth. This quickly produced monkeys that were severely disturbed, which were used as models of human depression. Harlow called the pit where the monkeys were held the 'well of despair'. He went on to suffer his own well of despair, and later in life was treated with electroconvulsive therapy for severe depression.

My bookshelves are filled with heavy, academic books, most of which I've sourced second-hand, giving my new nursing-home room the smell of an old library. I try and focus on the *Textbook of Paediatrics, Wong's Nursing Care of Infants and Children, The Colour Dictionary of Childhood Dermatology* (not recommended for the faint-hearted, or for my mum, who picked it up absent-mindedly one day and leafed through, only to not sleep a wink that night).

Ann Casey is an English nurse who developed Casey's Model of Nursing when she was working in paediatric oncology. Her theories are popular on children's wards, and all the documentation mentions family-centred care – the philosophy that the best people to care for a sick child are the parents or families or carers themselves, with the support of the nurses. In a recent interview she described the qualities of a good nurse as being inherently kind. But we have come a long way from what we originally thought 'kindness' means.

Children's nursing historically involved the discouragement of visits from family members, because it upset the children too greatly. Children were tied to their beds, sick and alone. Nowadays families are encouraged to be present throughout the entirety of their child's stay in hospital. There are makeshift camp beds next to the child's hospital bed, which we pull out for family members, and even a special accommodation unit in the hospital, designed for families of long-term sick children; these are often paid for with charity money, the nurses and doctors getting involved on their time off, raising money by walking 100 miles, climbing mountains, mega bike-rides. If the special accommodation is full, we send the parents of sick children to a nearby hotel where we have negotiated good rates. Unfortunately, this is central London, and the local sex workers apparently also enjoy good hotel rates. 'I kept getting knocks on the door from dubious-looking men looking for Patsy,' one parent reports back. 'And I do not want to tell you about the noises from next door.'

Of course it is not the books or academic theories that teach me how to nurse. I close my eyes and try and remember everything I learned in the classroom, from my books and libraries, and from nursing lecturers. Instead, what comes to mind is my time in hospital as a child, when I had pneumonia; and subsequent anaphylactic reactions to the antibiotics, and how my only sustaining memory from that time – aged eight, when I can well remember other incidents – is of a nurse who fed me orange yoghurt, very slowly, tiny spoonful after tiny spoonful. I remember nothing of the doctors who healed me, but I can still remember the taste of that orange yoghurt.

The London nursing students have double-barrelled surnames and long, flicky hair. There is only one man in my year, and he is the sole non-white nursing student. There have always been male nurses; in Alexandria in the third century AD male nurses were known as *parabalani*, meaning 'persons who risk their lives as nurses', due to their exposure to people with infectious diseases (the female nurses were not given such titles). During bouts of the plague in Europe, male nurses were the primary caregivers. In America, nursing schools for men were fairly common until the early 1900s, but by 1930 men constituted just 1 per cent of nurses. Unlike campaigns to increase and promote opportunities for women in medicine, there have been no such campaigns within nursing for men.

In some Francophile African countries – Chad, Cameroon, Guinea, Senegal and Rwanda, for example – there are more male nurses than female. And in European countries such as Spain, Italy and Portugal, 20 per cent of nurses are male. But in 2016 just 11.4 per cent of nurses in the UK were male. Much is written about the potential reasons for this, and about the idea that empathetic and caring traits are not exclusively feminine ones. But rather than excluding or discriminating against men, it could be argued that nursing is seen as one of the most lowly (female) professions there is, and therefore rather than integrating it along non-gender lines, the act of caring is not considered valuable. Female doctors are welcome in the club, but we, as nurses, are not promoting our club to male nurses – not because the men would not be welcome, but because of something deeper and far more disturbing. In my experience, the men I've worked with in nursing are fast-tracked to managerial positions. And research suggests that although there are far more women nurses, the comparatively few male nurses get paid more.

Student nurse Ismail lives with his wife and three children and he talks about them constantly. He will, I imagine, make a fantastic children's nurse. The rest of my class are twenty-something middle-class academic women from privileged backgrounds. It's a far cry from Bedford – where my cohort were diverse in age and race, and almost all from working-class families – despite being a short geographical distance away. And it's my first glimpse of the differences in nursing culture within a small part of London, even within different hospitals.

Each hospital is a country, unique and separate, with an infrastructure and philosophy different from the next one. In the hospital where I am working by now the nurses are slightly arrogant and generally old-fashioned. Always bossy. I have high hopes for my time here, though. It is the international home of cutting-edge paediatrics. If you want to learn how to nurse children, then surely this is the place. In 1918 Princess Mary trained at the children's hospital, Great Ormond Street. And in 1936 Princess Tsahai – the daughter of Emperor Haile Selassie – also completed her nursing training in London. She worked alongside the other student nurses for the required fifty-six hours a week and earned a year's salary of £20. She was taught to help others but died tragically at the age of just twenty-two years old, following a miscarriage, before she could put into practice all she had learned.

I imagine Princess Tsahai (she was described as dignified and graceful) and stand taller, vowing to make the most not only of the second half of my training, but also of the opportunities that living in central London will give me access to:

culture, fine restaurants, theatre, opera, ballet and art. But I don't manage dignity or style. Instead, we second-year student nurses down electric-blue cocktails and flaming sambucas at a local dive-bar and gossip about lovers. We drink too much. When my dad comes to visit and brings his neighbour to help move the rest of my things in, I am sick on his shoes in the passenger seat of a borrowed van. 'Bloody students!' he says, dismissing my nurse's cape, and hat and belt buckle, and my protests that it must have been something I ate.

I am sent for my first ever paediatrics placement to Hackney Road, which we call – pre-hipster bars and regeneration – 'Murder Mile'. The hospital in east London is local and, although it is affiliated with the tertiary and specialist children's hospital where most of my training takes place, it is a world away. I have my uniform neatly pressed, my belt buckle shining, my fob watch pinned to my collar, a selection of pens in my pocket; my shoes are new, squeaky and shiny – I am ready.

Within two weeks I have scabies, impetigo and nits. I've been bitten by a child and had to have a hepatitis booster; and I have had an 'eye washout', after a baby who was having a nappy change had explosive diarrhoea all over my face. I was expecting cutting-edge paediatrics. Instead, I find myself spending much of my time caring for children who are consti-pated, needing bowel washouts following poor diets; who have rickets due to lack of vitamin D; who have needed all their teeth taken out, after drinking Coca-Cola from a baby bottle for two years; who are severely malnourished ('failure to thrive') or on fat-reducing diets; or who have measles, as they did not get the MMR immunisation, and now have serious complications as a result of contracting the illness. I find out that the acronym FLK stands simply for 'funny-looking kid'. It's like living in a Dickens novel; indeed, Dickens was instrumental in saving another London children's hospital from financial ruin, by speaking at a festival dinner and giving a public reading of *A Christmas Carol*.

'Sorry,' I say during handover. 'What do you mean? I'm not sure I understand the diagnosis.' We are huddled in the staffroom, frantically scribbling information down on scraps of paper. The walls are lined with out-of-date information. Everything about the room is tired: the chairs sagging and breaking, a plant in the corner of another coffee room long dead. The bin in the corner is overflowing with Hula Hoop crisp packets and empty plastic coffee cups. Everything smells of feet and beef-flavouring.

The matron in charge narrows her eyes at me. She's a fierce, skinny Irish woman who has the reputation of going round the hospital in the middle of the night, touching the televisions with the palms of her hands. God help any nurses whose television is warm. I see her do it once, and it looks almost spiritual – her arms stretched out before her, fingertips spread out, hands pressing into the screen; she kneels in front of the TV, as if praying.

'I'm sorry,' I repeat, 'are they diabetic?' My mind runs over all the books I've studied, and I can't remember any mention of fat-reducing treatment. I search in my mind for information about childhood diseases: glandular fever; febrile convulsions; diabetes; bronchiolitis; appendicitis; intussusception; sickle-cell anaemia; nephrotic syndrome; croup; haemophilia; cystic fibrosis.

I scratch my head. The nits have returned, despite constant washing of my now-brittle and dry hair with tea-tree oil. Everything itches. I have ringworm too, on my forearm – a round, white raised area, like a miniature crop circle.

'Fat-reducing diets,' she says, lowering her glasses to the end of her nose and peering at me over the top, 'are diets for fat children.'

I remember a condition called Prader–Willi syndrome that I've read about, and I am about to question her again. I open my mouth to speak, but she silences me with a skeletal waving hand. I close my mouth.

'Nothing medical here, at the moment. All social,' she says. 'The children are fat. Dangerously fat. Enormously fat. Hence the fat-reducing diets. Or they are constipated, due to a different kind of bad diet. Or they have emotional problems, mental-health problems, or are here for long-term bed-wetting. Anxiety, anorexia, OCD, ADHD, depression –

you name it.' She pushes her glasses up onto her nose and squeezes her thin lips together. 'We see all manner of child abuse, too, on the children's ward. And not only here. All hospitals, across the board. You are not in Kansas any more, my dear,' she says.

There are quite a few children that I care for during the placement who are simply fat. Globally, the World Health Organization states that in 2015 the number of overweight children under the age of five was estimated to be more than forty-two million. In the UK approximately 10 per cent of children are obese. And these figures are rising.

I spend my first day watching for smuggled-in KFC or hidden burger wrappers, and for things being thrown around the ward by a thirteen-year-old boy called Jerome, who has challenging behaviour as well as sickle-cell disease and is on a morphine infusion to reduce the pain. I look after a fat baby with asthma wearing a neon-green string vest, with a continuous caterpillar of snot hanging over his smiling mouth. 'Happy wheezer, we call them,' says the nurse in charge. 'Well, get on and wipe him clean, then.'

Children's nurses have to be child-whisperers, able to communicate with children who are frightened and in pain. They remind us of something that Florence Nightingale herself knew. Suffering, and even the sensation of pain, can be reduced by kindness. She found that giving a patient a window to look out of, or a bunch of flowers, will significantly affect their experience of illness. Children in hospital need to play. Play is the work – and therapy – of childhood. So play therapists are vital. At the time I am learning to nurse children, my mum is becoming a therapeutic social worker. She shows me photographs of her playroom, and her sandpit and children's artwork, and describes how she can read a child's painting as a clairvoyant reads tea leaves, or can look at the mess a child has made in a sandpit and predict their future.

But sometimes a window or flowers, or even opportunities for play, are difficult to provide. Rohan is a four-year-old boy with Severe Combined Immunodeficiency Disorder. This is a group of rare, sometimes fatal genetic conditions, characterised by little or no immune response to infection. This leaves the patient unable to fight infections, viruses and bacteria. We called them the 'SCID kids', but these children are also said to have 'Bubble Boy syndrome', after David Vetter, who lived in a plastic germ-free bubble until he died, aged twelve. When Vetter was four years old he discovered that he could poke holes in the bubble with a syringe that was accidentally left in his room; later, when NASA designed a special suit to enable him to leave the house, he used it only seven times, and when he outgrew it, he didn't use the new one at all.

Rohan does not live in a bubble, thanks to laminar airflow rooms and advanced technology, but his airlocked room, minimal visitors and a small selection of toys are still his entire life. And his life is intensely lonely. He looks at the world through glass windows, and waves every now and then at the nurses passing by. His wave is not enthusiastic, though. His arm flaps slowly and awkwardly. He is developmentally delayed and small for his age. Rohan's parents – as is common with the families of disabled children – are long separated. They take turns visiting. His mother spends a long time outside the room, getting updates from the nurses about Rohan's condition. His father strides straight in through the airlock doors (the area between Rohan's room and the outside world, where the air is cleaned), washes his hands, then bounds into the room, picking Rohan up and throwing him in the air a bit. I try and stand nearby whenever the father arrives, knowing that the highlight of my day will be seeing the expression on Rohan's face as his dad lifts him up. He comes to life for a short time. He is poking through his bubble with a leftover syringe.

It is amazing, and sad, what can become normal. Rohan has blood tests so often that he never cries. He holds his arm out and lets the doctors take blood at any time. The nurses are busy and often, after the long hand-washing process to change his nappy, due to his constant watery diarrhoea, there is no time to play. His dry eyes are the saddest thing ever. Being so sick does not excuse Rohan from hospital school, though. The hospital has a fully functioning school. Children push their drip-stands, or can be brought in wheelchairs, to the classrooms with the teacher. Of course these are very special teachers. If the children are too sick to leave their beds, or are on dialysis machines, hooked up and twisted around technology like hostages tied up with tubing, then the teachers visit their beds, sit for a while and set them some work to do. 'Education and health are one and the same. A basic human right. A child in hospital should have more than the basic human rights honoured,' a hospital teacher tells me.

Rohan's mum is arguing with the teachers about germs. She feels that it is not in his interests for a different person, as well as a nurse, to go in and out of his room every day, when he is so close to a bone-marrow transplant. Every time somebody goes in, he is at risk, no matter how well people wash their hands. 'The risk is too great,' she says. 'And he will not miss a few weeks more, with everything else he has missed. He's only four for heaven's sake. Reception class doesn't matter.'

I understand that Rohan's mum is a lioness and will protect him above all else. That is her job. Yet it's hard not to think of the NASA-designed suit for David Vetter, which was meant to allow freedom, but over time got used less and less. Rohan may have more chances of survival by living in a bubble, with extremely limited exposure to people. But at what cost? Later, though, I hear that Rohan's bone-marrow transplant was successful and he made it home. I like to think of him in the park, on a bike, with the sun and wind on his face.

*

'There is a spider in my head.' Tia is five years old and has the ear of a soft toy rabbit in her mouth as she speaks. Her aunt, Caroline, is sitting next to her. Her parents have gone off the ward, after speaking to the doctors. Both of them are crying.

'Tia, you know it's not a real spider.' Caroline half-smiles at me, but the smile doesn't reach her eyes.

I kneel in front of Tia. 'The type of lump in your head looks exactly like a spider,' I say. 'I know what you mean.'

Tia has been diagnosed with an aggressive astrocytoma, a type of brain tumour that is in a difficult place. She is due to have surgery, followed by chemotherapy and radiotherapy. 'She was vomiting every morning,' Caroline tells me. 'Projectile vomiting. And complaining that her eyes didn't work, so we figured she was having blurred vision. The GP referred us, and then suddenly we are here.'

'It's definitely a spider,' says Tia. 'Rabbit thinks so, too.' She takes the chewed-up ear out of her mouth. Her eyes are wider than the moon. She looks straight up at me and whispers, 'They want to take it out.'

I try to smile and not let my voice wobble, but Caroline covers her mouth with her hand and makes a terrible sound.

I am finally qualified as a children's nurse. I am twenty years old and still have my shining fob watch that I used on my first day as a student, but my shoes no longer squeak, my immune system has been exposed to so many infections that I have built up defences against all kinds of bacteria, viruses and fungi. I am lucky enough to have an immune system that works much better than Rohan's, protecting me. My physical health is perfect. Still, I am terrified. Pumpkin Ward, where I've secured my first job as a qualified nurse, is a place of high risk. The babies and children are having spinal surgery, neuro-surgery and craniofacial surgery.

After putting on a Disney film for Tia, and my arm around Caroline, I check on my other patient, Joseph.

'When he was born, we didn't get a single Congratulations card. Not from colleagues, and not even from family. Imagine that?' Joseph's mum, Deborah, is a too-thin woman with bitten-down nails and unruly hair tied up in a knot on top of her head, a cup of coffee in her hand. I wonder when she last had time to look after herself. Joseph suffers from Nager syndrome, a rare genetic disorder, and has an almost missing jaw. He's receiving jaw reconstruction and is on his fifth surgery. He's nine years old.

'ENT are involved, but don't want to tracheotomy him again,' she says. She slips in and out of medical terminology and language that does not, and should not, belong to the mother of a child, a layperson who has spent too long around doctors. The words get mixed up and come out wrong, as though she has taken an advanced language class without the basic beginning section.

'I didn't realise he'd had a tracheostomy. Is he your first?' I ask.

'First and last,' she says. 'Joseph needs all my attention. I've gone part-time, but it's busy. Well, you know busy.'

I don't know. Not yet. It's only my second day as a qualified nurse and I feel as if I know nothing at all. But I don't mention that; I don't want to add to her nerves. There is so much to learn. Along with Nager syndrome, there are dozens of other genetic abnormalities and strange syndromes at this hospital. One student-nurse friend comments that we only see the 'weird and wonderful' conditions here.

I am in the tertiary centre, which provides specialised care and rare treatments that are not available at local hospitals, meaning that patients come from all over the country (50 per cent from London) and internationally. It is almost impossible to know them all, but I stay up late into the night learning about the frequency of genetic abnormalities in the consanguineous families (first cousins who marry) that we see in London, or memorising the names and symptoms of syndromes: Metopic Craniosynostosis; Apert syndrome; Plagiocephaly; Pfeiffer syndrome; Fibrous Dysplasia; Carpenter syndrome.

I have a book of photographs of some of the craniofacial conditions, and I discover that Freeman–Sheldon syndrome used to be called 'Whistling-face syndrome', as the children are born with underdeveloped mouths and pursed lips and appear to be whistling. I show the photograph to a doctor friend, who says, 'In Egypt, in the village I am from, we would leave these children out to die.'

I find that my friends are all becoming doctors, nurses and midwives, and my non-nursing friends are dropping off. One who works in an office complains all the time about her difficult day. Another complains that his baby's crying is worrying him so much, there might be something wrong. 'Really sick babies don't cry,' I say. I have decreasing sympathy for normal problems. Friends I grew up with ask about nursing. 'It's hard to explain,' I tell them. 'You are changing,' they tell me.

'Christie, can you come and check the bed space in the High-Dependency Unit?' Anna, the sister, pokes her head into the room. She is wearing an old-fashioned dark-blue nurse's dress. The sleeves have a perfectly starched crease in the sides.

'I'll see you later,' I say to Deborah. I turn to Joseph: 'And you, little man.' I am conscious of the amount of time my eyes fall on his face. He has such an unusual face, sharp and pointed and squished together, that it is difficult not to look, not to stare. I can't imagine what it must be like for him, for his mum, to be constantly reminded of the difference. He gives me a big smile, and his face is beautiful at once.

I follow Anna down the corridor. I'll be shadowing Anna, looking after Joseph post-operatively. Orientation to my new ward, and being newly qualified, means following around the experienced nurses for anything from a few days to a few months, in order to learn the ropes, and for the experienced nurse to check that the rookie is safe to let loose on patients.

'We'll have to get an emergency trachy, but there are oropharangeal airways there, next to the bed.'

I look at the three tubes next to the bed, much smaller than they should be, adapted to fit Joseph's face.

'If he stops breathing, don't press the face-mask down too hard, or his face will collapse. Insert a Guedel first.'

I nod and feel my eyes widening, the burning of sick in my throat. I swallow hard and try to breathe slowly. Her voice doesn't change a note as she says 'or his face will collapse'. There is no pause or deep breath, or arm on my shoulder. It is a matter of fact.

Anna laughs. 'You'll be fine,' she says. 'I'm here.' She has worked on the paediatric neurosurgical unit for years. She is an old-school nurse, immaculate and matronly, wearing her sharply ironed dress and a fob watch, which she glances at as she talks. She's studying for a PhD in an obscure neurosurgical condition, and her office is bursting with scientific papers that she encourages the other nurses to read, if the ward is not busy, instead of the magazines that are piled up underneath the desk. It's her day off today, but one of the rostered student nurses is attending a family friend's funeral. 'I'm not sure if I'm allowed a compassionate day, because it's not direct family,' she had said, to which Anna had replied that the day when nurses are not compassionate towards each other will herald the end of things. 'It's fine. Take as long as you need. I'll cover you.'

I follow Anna around like a lost puppy and try to memorise everything. She does everything – from cleaning a dirty toilet rather than wait for the cleaner, 'in case the parents want to use it', to arguing with the neurosurgeons about treatment plans, holding up scans and pointing to strange, swirling patterns that make no sense at all to me, explaining that the foramen magnum decompression operation – while necessary if the child develops further breathing problems – is not warranted, based on a worrying-looking scan alone. She explains to me afterwards, 'We treat the whole patient, and the family, and don't simply use the scan. We are not performing unnecessary surgeries in order to generate income.' She sighs. 'Not yet anyway. We still have an NHS.'

The junior doctors all want to be around Anna, listening – as I do – to her approach to everything, her knowledge echoing out into the corridors. But Anna is more interested in the nurses. There is a low turnover on the ward and the nurses stay for years; some of them a lifetime.

'Check the bed space, and then double-check. I'll be here, but I want to see that you can manage.' She talks as she walks in front of me, without turning her head. She knows I will follow.

I try and place my steps beside Anna's, matching her stride, copying her straight posture, her head flicking from side to side as she walks, glancing at each room, assessing the cleanliness, the danger, sensory details that tell her the ward is ship-shape: the quiet buzzing of the drugs fridges, the squeak of her shoes on the well-polished floor, the quiet of the parents and their children in each side-room.

There is a bathroom opposite the kitchen, with a bath for the children, and a hoist to get in and out of the bath for the children who can't stand. Usually, though, we lift them – a practice I'll regret later on. Around the corner is the nurses' station, a square-shaped area separated by desks, behind which is an X-ray board, a notes trolley and shelving containing thick reference books and plastic files; a single computer on the desk and two telephones; as well as a small, square white alarm, which flashes orange if any of the relatives pull the call bell, and red if they pull the emergency bell. There is also the area where we lay out snacks during the night shift: bowls of sweets that the families leave for us, crisps, a tray of chicken that the agency nurse from the Czech Republic tells us is her grandmother's recipe.

Opposite the nurses' station is the high-dependency area, then a long, thin ward with single rooms, all with a bathroom and a pull-out bed, allowing a parent to stay with their child in the hospital. The other side of the nurses' station is the treatment room, filled with equipment, where the doctors insert drips into (cannulate) children; or the nurses unwrap children's heads from bandages, pull out staples or stitches from their skull, while the play therapist, Malin, kneels in front of them, blowing bubbles. There is a staffroom next door and a doctor's office, where multidisciplinary team meetings take place to decide treatment regimes and discuss morbidity and mortality; and – on the arrival of a staff member's baby, or when someone leaves to move to another ward or hospital – to have tea and a variety of cakes.

The drugs room is a long, thin room next door. Each eye-height cupboard contains stacks of different medications, checked every day by a pharmacist who comes to each ward with a clipboard and checklist. There is a large stack of transparent plastic trays piled up at the end, next to the sink that we use for drawing up intravenous and, occasionally, intrathecal drugs (which are injected straight into the spinal fluid, thereby negating the need for the drug to cross the blood–brain barrier).

We stop at the four-bed high-dependency area opposite the nurses' station. Each nurse will care for two children and, although this is not intensive care, occasionally the anaesthetists will bring the children back to this area, on the ward, even if they need ventilating, arguing that the specialist nature of the neurosurgical nurses and doctors represents a safer place for these children than a general Intensive-Care Unit. I am a junior, but already I appreciate how terrifying a place this is for a newly qualified nurse. I look at the list of patients on the whiteboard and try not to panic, thinking about the conditions these children suffer from that bring them to need neurosurgery in our ward, which accepts children from birth to eighteen years old: intractable epilepsy, hydrocephalus, brain tumours, spinal-cord injuries, aneurisms, strokes, neurofibromatosis, tethered spinal-cord syndrome. It's hard not to feel anxious.

My hands are flaky, sore and dry, from the number of times I am washing them, covering them in alcohol gel, cleaning bed spaces with alcohol wipes and disinfectant. On Pumpkin Ward, due to the nature of the surgery, the infection the children are at risk of is meningitis. I've already been tasked with the lumber-puncture test, to assess a child for infection. This involves curling a child up like a comma, and keeping them completely still, while the doctor inserts a large needle directly into the spinal cavity, to collect cerebrospinal fluid to check for infection markers and assess the pressure. The job of the doctor relies on extreme technical skill. The nurse's job is less well defined. Keeping a toddler or a child completely still and calm, curled over for a painful procedure, is tricky, and any tiny movement is potentially dangerous. It relies on knowledge about that particular child.

Ahmed, two years old, loves Donald Duck, so an ability to imitate Donald's voice, and an understanding that telling a story in the right way – with the exciting part revealed at the exact moment to capture his attention and distract him from what's going on in his back – is useful. Then there's Sharlini, aged eleven, who has severe disabilities and can jerk suddenly without any reason. After I have spent days with the family, her mum tells me that Sharlini can keep perfectly still during the introduction of Prince's 'Little Red Corvette'. Before the procedure, I find the CD player, pause it at the exact point and make sure the volume is at the right level, while the doctor scrubs his hands, my thumb poised over the play button.

Throughout it all, Anna remains calm. There is a time – a kind of calm before the storm – when the children are pre-theatre, and I wash everything down, again, with soapy water and then alcohol wipes; check the oxygen, suction, monitors; make sure the bag valve mask and oropharangeal airways are close to hand; and pray quietly that Joseph doesn't stop breathing post-operatively.

'Get yourself some tea and toast,' Anna says. 'You'll be fine. I'm here.'

I go into the small ward kitchen, where there is an urn that we put on every morning to keep water boiling, rather than wait precious seconds for the kettle to boil; a dishwasher; a giant tub of Nescafé and, sometimes, in-date milk in the fridge. There's a toaster, too, although there is talk of having it taken away, as the fire brigade has to come out every time the smoke alarm goes off for burnt toast.

The cleaner, Bola, comes in while I'm making some coffee. She is a larger-than-life, happy woman who I've never seen not smiling. 'Christie, your second day. How is it being a qualified nurse?'

'Scary.' I smile.

'Aha, well, I have some dried prawns for you.' She unlocks the cupboard, then rummages around and pulls out her battered brown handbag. She passes me a foil-wrapped package, inside which are what look like chilli peppers, but are actually dried fish.

I laugh. Try one. Cough. 'Thanks.'

I leave Bola as she begins washing up; she doesn't believe in dishwashers, she says, as she turns back to the sink and starts singing a church song. I want to hide in the kitchen with her all day, eating spicy food and listening to her voice.

Joseph arrives back on the ward, covered in bandages. His mum stands next to his bed, while I write down his observations and watch Anna as she gives him an injection of pain relief. He is stable, and the tubes next to him remain unused. After only a few hours he sits up and sips some water through a straw. 'My little fighter,' his mum says.

I follow Anna to the main ward area and to bed eight, where Anna has asked me to give my first intramuscular injection, to a fifteen-year-old who needs codeine phosphate for pain, following spinal surgery. I copy her actions on Joseph, finding the landmarks of the boy's outer thigh and inserting the needle into his muscle, pulling back a tiny amount to make sure there is no blood returning into the syringe, indicating that I've hit a vein; on seeing it clear, I inject the fluid. My nerves make my hands shake. We practised various injection techniques as students, but on fake limbs and oranges. Once, we even practised on each other, cannulating and inserting nasogastric tubes. 'If you can't stomach the thought of it on yourself, imagine how terrible it is for the poor children you will be caring for.'

Injecting into a real person – a patient, a child – is far scarier. Anna is behind me the entire time. I look back and she nods at every stage. At the very last minute I begin to draw the needle out and my arm jerks violently. The needle snaps off, half in my hand with the syringe, and half inside his leg muscle.

'Oh my God,' I say. 'Oh my God!'

I feel Anna's hand on the small of my back. 'Keep calm. It's not a problem.' She has an apron and gloves on in seconds and whips the needle out between her fingers, dropping it into the sharps bin as though it were a piece of fluff or a stray hair on the boy's jumper. He smiles. Anna smiles. I burst into tears.

We walk into the coffee room and I can't stop crying. Anna has her arm around me.

'You have to make mistakes,' she says. 'You're a perfectionist, and you can't be perfect in your first job. Or ever.'

She laughs. 'I make mistakes all the time. I know a nurse who cut through a child's external ventricular drain, you know? Imagine that! Cerebrospinal fluid dripping out. It was a serious problem. We fixed it. And other things happen that you can't predict. Philippe bit through his Hickman line last week and nearly bled to death in his cot. If I hadn't gone in to do a set of obs, who knows what would have happened.' She squeezes my arm. 'But there was no harm done.'

The sixteenth-century French Renaissance philosopher Michel de Montaigne was obsessed with what being human means. He described doctors as having the advantage that 'the sun lights their success and the earth covers their failures'. I already know there is a difference in the way nurses are treated following a mistake – differently from their medical counterparts. 'We don't stick up for each other in the way that doctors do,' says a colleague, after a child is given a drug intrathecally that travels straight into the spinal canal or into the subarachnoid space, instead of intravenously, with devastating consequences. A simple thing. Right drug, right patient, right dose; wrong method of administration. 'It will be the nurse who gets struck off, for carrying the drug to the doctors, I'll bet, not the doctors who administered it.' But I can also tell that Anna will treat nurses and doctors exactly the same, not covering their mistakes, but acknowledging that we are, after all, human; and learning; and sometimes we are sorry.

My immune system may be robust, but my emotional immunity is incredibly fragile.

'It was my first injection,' I say. 'I'm going to be a rubbish nurse.'

'Nonsense,' Anna says. 'All my nurses are excellent.'

On night shifts there are usually fewer nurses, as there is less work to do, but on the neurosurgical ward the intravenous drugs are administered regularly and we wake up children often, to perform neurological observations, using the Glasgow Coma Scale, which was developed in order to check a patient's responsiveness and conscious level. If a child is not responding to a voice, the nurse must squeeze the trapezius muscle between the neck and shoulder to see if the child responds normally, ensuring that the doctors do not try any methods of painful stimuli that they learned when such things were considered acceptable: rubbing the child's sternum with their knuckles, pressing a pen on a child's fingernail or twisting their ear.

'The child may well feel pain, but be unable to respond,' Anna says. 'So if you see a doctor using old barbaric methods of torture, then stop them.' She tells me that the Glasgow Coma Scale is important, but there are other neurological signs and symptoms that the chart does not recognise, although her nurses must: a child who hiccups regularly, has a change of tone, becomes stiff or floppy, has a tense or bulging fontanelle, vomits, shows sun-setting eyes or has a parent or caregiver who reports a change. 'Always trust the mother,' she says. 'The mother knows her child better than us, better than any consultant in the world. If the mother says something is wrong with her daughter or son, then you believe her. And the other thing to look for, of course, is yawning.'

I find that I have covered my mouth with my hand in a poor attempt to suppress a yawn, which bursts out anyway. It is busy on the ward and I'm pretty useless; nervous and tired, unused to night work and almost unable to keep my eyes from closing.

'You can have a sleep shortly, a little break, but there's an emergency coming in – query blocked shunt – and I want you to do fifteen-minute neuro-obs.'

The ward accepts blocked shunts regardless of whether they have space. They make space. These are classed as neuro-surgical emergencies. A ventricular peritoneal shunt is one of the treatments for hydrocephalus, or what is sometimes called 'water on the brain', the babies who come in with giant, alien-looking heads, eyes bulging downwards as the pressure is so great. My orientation included some time in theatre, and I had to leave during a shunt operation. It is brutal surgery, clunky and messy. I understood the procedure, and the drilling of the skull part wasn't as bad as I'd imagined: a colleague had warned me about the smell of burnt toast. But I hadn't imagined how it would feel to see the catheter being pushed in and threaded into the brain, the other catheter pushed from behind the ear into the chest, then the stomach, where the excess fluid is reabsorbed by the child's body. I hadn't imagined how much effort it would take the surgeon to push a tube through a scrap of a body. The child with the 'query blocked shunt' has been coming in every four out of five months with shunt issues. The surgery has a high failure rate, but is essential nonetheless. Without it, the child will die. It is 3 a.m. when she finally goes down to theatre. The neurosurgeons and theatre team have been called from home. It can't wait until morning.

In the meantime, I go and check on Tia, who is fast asleep and cuddling her small purple rabbit. I don't wake her. She doesn't need observations as regularly, although she has the tumour in her head. There is something particularly horrifying about a child with a brain tumour. Maybe because they look so well and, in treating them, they become so ill. Or because it reminds us that life is completely random, and our lack of ability to control nature is terrifying. No parent should ever have to face what Tia's parents are facing.

I sit down by the nurses' station. Anna walks past and sees me sitting. 'Have a sleep. Just lie down in the doctor's office.'

'No,' I say, 'I'm okay. I'm sorry – just haven't sat down all night.'

'Look, we all do it. And it's better if you go now...' She's walking away while she speaks and there's a queue of people waiting to get her attention, ask her questions or advice about drug doses or admissions or staffing issues.

I enter the code for the office door that I've scribbled on the back of my hand. Inside is a small neat office, a desk and computer, a wall-chart calendar and a small couch. I won't have been the first to use it to sleep on. There is a cushion and a folded-up sheet hanging over the arm. A coat hanger is on the back of the door, with a hook. I look down at my dress, starched and immaculate. I spent a long time ironing my uniform with starch, spraying the collar. I even polished my silver belt buckle. There is no way I'm getting it creased. I check and double-check that the door is locked, then take off my dress, hang it up and brush it down, before climbing onto the couch and wrapping myself in the sheet.

I wake to laughter. There are three or four male doctors standing above me. 'Erm, good morning,' one of them says. 'I'm Dr Barnes.' He is wearing a pinstripe suit, a stethoscope around his neck, is carrying a briefcase and looks important. I am unable to move or speak for many minutes. It is morning – bright light and daytime sounds: the kitchen staff clattering plates, the sound of children crying, people talking, a radio. Gradually I realise where I am, and see my dress hanging on the back of the door. I feel as if I am in a *Carry On* film.

'I'm so sorry,' I say, pulling the sheet up to my chin. 'I'm so sorry.' I turn my head away, to hide the face full of redness that I know I have. 'I'm sorry. They must have forgotten me. I'm new. I didn't want to get my dress creased.'

It doesn't take long until I hardly recognise myself. It is impossible to describe exactly what I learn, though I know it lies somewhere between science and art. It is all about the smallest details, and understanding how they make the biggest difference.

Today I'm caring for four children. The first has an external ventricular drain to measure cerebrospinal fluid. In the next bed is Tia, who will be going for radiotherapy later today. She had her surgery some time ago, but the cancer came back. Now it is time for her second round of chemo-therapy and radiotherapy. The other two children are an eight-year-old boy who suffers with neurofibromatosis and has autism, and a ten-year-old girl with severe epilepsy, who is due to have surgery the following day. I talk and listen to a dad whose child is going to have half her brain removed – an operation called a hemispherectomy – for intractable epilepsy. She needs plenty of pre-operation paperwork, care-planning documentation filling in and blood tests. 'It's like Frankenstein,' her dad says. He's a stocky truck driver with tattoos covering his knuckles. He talks about football (Arsenal) and nips in and out of the hospital all day to smoke roll-up cigarettes. 'They're basically cutting out half her brain to stop the fits.'

Brain surgery to treat epilepsy is not a new idea. In South America, pre-Incan civilisations drilled burr holes and removed pieces of skull, using surgical tools made of bronze and sharp-edged volcanic rock, to treat spiritual and magical problems, as well as headaches, epilepsy and mental illness. Of course surgery has developed hugely since the early days and it represents only one way of treating epilepsy. Most people with severe epilepsy can manage their illness successfully on anti-epileptic drugs. But the small percentage of people who have such severe epilepsy that they are willing to have dangerous surgery – which at best produces a 70 per cent success rate – are usually so disabled by their constant fitting that there really is no alternative. And for a few in that lucky 70 per cent the seizures may stop altogether. But epilepsy seizures are not one thing or another. There are as many different kinds as there are different kinds of winds, all with their own origin, language and outcome. The hemispherectomy which the dad describes to me will mean that his daughter is left paralysed down one side of her body like a person following a stroke; and although her type of seizures, called 'drop attacks', will stop (meaning that she won't have to wear a helmet and suffer head injury after head injury), she might have more frequent seizures of a different nature. Surgery can change a weather pattern, but only nature can change the weather itself.

It is Tia who is taking up most of my time, though she is currently the least critically sick child in my care. She is in the playroom when I look for her to do a set of neurological observations. She's playing with what I first think is Play-Doh, but which Malin, the play therapist, tells me is the substance from the mould-room that they use to make Tia's radiotherapy mask. Her purple rabbit lies on the table. 'She needs to have the mask fitted over her entire face and head. Then they'll use it when she has radiotherapy, basically screw it into the trolley so that she can't move an inch or speak. The laser needs to be exact, and not a millimetre out.'

I know this already, but I am in awe of a child brave enough to go through it. I try to imagine having a hard mask over my entire face, pinning me down so that I can't move. It's hard even to think about it. 'How will she tolerate it? Surely they'll have to give her a general anaesthetic?'

'She's six now, so it's borderline, but much better not to. Play therapy is the best option.'

Malin is not a nurse, and she is poorly paid. Her skills are often overlooked by the surgeons. Yet she can counsel a six-year-old through treatment for brain cancer, and can distract a child from extreme pain. Her understanding and knowledge of child development make an enormous differ-ence to a child's level of suffering and the memory of that experience. The child will not remember the surgeon who saved his or her life, but will always remember Malin, who blew the bubbles. The child remembers the clown doctor who visits and performs magic tricks. And the yellow Labrador brought to the hospital by the pet charity. And the lady from the hospital radio who performs a shout-out to 'Millie in bed ten on ward seven'. Plus the volunteer who brings Harry Potter books on a small trolley.

But Tia is not smiling. She holds the Play-Doh-type mask between her fingertips, without making anything for a while. She has the face of an old woman, twisted and worried, despite being only six years old. 'Be brave, Softie,' she says to the rabbit, repeatedly putting the mould on its face, then quickly pulling it off, picking the rabbit up and kissing it. 'Be brave.'

When it is time to take Tia downstairs to have the mask fitted, she screams in such a way that I can hear it inside my bones. Tia is physically strong. Her immune system has yet to be damaged by the treatment she so desperately needs. It's hard to imagine her in the state that she was in after her last treatment: weakened, unable to move or talk, with a mouth full of ulcers from infections that her damaged immune system could not fight. Hard to imagine that this is our aim, again. I do not want to think about her cancer coming back, and what it might mean for her chances. For now, her body fights. And my own emotional immunity is building up. I hear her scream as if from far away. I have a job to do, and crying will not help. Tia arches her back and becomes stiff and impossible to pick up. We have to postpone the fitting, let her mum hold her and rock her until the screaming diminishes.

I am leaving Pumpkin Ward for a promotion: to work in the community as an assistant manager in a respite centre for severely disabled children. The nurses congratulate me. The doctors congratulate me. The children and families congratulate me. On my last day there is cake and tea in the large office, with various scans of brain tumours lining the walls instead of art. I try not to look at Tia's scan, but my eyes keep rolling towards it – the impossibly large, white spider in the centre of the picture. My colleagues take my mind off it. They chat and give me cards and hugs. But something is off. Everyone smiles a little too long. Some of my colleagues nip in and out of the bedrooms of the children that I'm caring for. Anna leaves early. Before going, she hugs me tightly and quickly. There is no emotion in her face, but I feel like holding onto her and never letting go.

'Thank you for being my mentor' is all I can manage to say. I want to say much, much more. How I hope some day to be like her. That she has taught me kindness and teamwork and professionalism; how to be hard and soft at the same time. That I will always be grateful to her. Anna has taught me how to be a nurse. After three years of training, my learning to be a nurse really began on my first day after I qualified.

But I still have no language to describe what I've learned from Anna. And she's already rushing away.

'Come along, Christie,' she says. 'Your shift isn't over yet. You are still one of my A-Team, and bed six needs attention.'

My colleagues shout for help from the bathroom. I run, imagining a child having a seizure or cardiac arrest, but when I get there, they are laughing. They throw me into a bath full of mushroom soup. It is revolting. The smell makes me retch and my skin absorbs the stickiness straight away. I try and jump out, but fall back in. How my colleagues have found enough soup to fill a bath, I'll never know. It's in my nose, in my hair, in my mouth: cold mushroom soup. There is silence for a few seconds, the cold shock of the bath. Then there is loud laughter.

There is a crowd congregating outside the bathroom, looking in. I have never heard a sound so beautiful as the laughter of those children gathered round in their wheelchairs or holding drip-stands – the faces of half a dozen children, each peering over and round to get a better look at me. Tia stands right at the front. She points right at me and laughs from her belly, the echo of it filling the bathroom. She laughs and laughs and laughs. She lies down on the floor in the doorway and rolls. Laughing and laughing and laughing. It makes everybody else laugh.

The doctors come out of the office and stand behind the children. Bola comes from the kitchen. The nurses come from next door. They glance at me covered in soup, but it is Tia everyone is watching. I find that I, too, am laughing. Laughing full belly-laughs for the first time in a long time, perhaps since Callum's suicide. A nurse–patient relationship is a two-way process, and Tia's laughter is infectious enough that it breaks through any of my self-inflicted emotional immunity. Her laughter makes me better. We can both cry, and we can both laugh. It is a beautiful sound. Her mum stands over Tia, smiles at me and opens and closes her hand, as if she is trying to capture the noise and keep hold of it for ever. I do the same.

'Remember, remember, remember,' I tell myself. Nursing requires building immunity to sorrow, but nursing children also requires being silly. Being chucked in a bath full of soup. Making a child laugh. Nursing means recognising that when there is a large white cloud at the centre of her child's scan, a mother needs something important to hold onto.

5

The Struggle for Existence

Give me a child until he is seven and I will show you the man.

Aristotle

The very best thing about being a children's nurse is that part of my job is cuddling babies. I love working in special care. The Neonatal Intensive-Care Unit (NICU) that also houses the Special-Care Baby Unit (SCBU) is the area of the hospital that admits premature babies, plus babies immediately from birth. Most of the babies here are teeny-tiny scraps of things, simply born too soon. Some of them spend many months here, and have various complications of prematurity. I once looked after a baby who had spent more than a year on a special-care unit and was still newborn-sized.

All NICUs have coded doors: women try to steal babies from hospitals. There's a blurry photograph on the wall of the coffee room of a woman identified as a risk, with text from the security department to accompany the photograph: 'If you see this woman, please contact security immediately. She is considered dangerous and has tried to enter wards disguised as a nurse.' I often stare at the photograph while I drink my morning coffee and wonder about her story, what led her to such desperation.

I enter the code for the door and push it open with a heavy click; immediately I'm confronted by the sour tang of breast milk, along with a blast of overwhelming heat. The unit is kept hot all year round. I'm glad of the loose cotton scrubs I wear (instead of the thicker nurse's dress worn in other wards) and the clogs, which allow my feet to breathe. I walk past fridges containing mainly drugs, past the transparent cupboard filled with drawers of consumables: bandages, needles, stickers, cardboard trays, endotracheal tubes, suction catheters, dressings, miniature woollen hats (knitted mostly by retired volunteer women, many of whom are ex-nurses from organisations with grand titles, such as the League of Nurses). There are noticeboards with information about research and doctors' rotas, and a large section of wall is taken up with Thank You cards:

We stayed in the unit for five months. It was the longest five months ever but, thanks to the nurses' humour and kindness, we kept our sanity!

Thank you to Carol, Mo and the team for putting up with my husband's jokes (and for SAVING the lives of our twin boys).

For the doctors and nurses of special care. We will never forget you.

To Maddie, the bereavement midwife. You helped us through the worst time of our life. We will treasure the memories you let us make during Annabelle's short time. Thank you is not enough. But there are no words.

A locked drugs cupboard stands next to the Thank You cards, with a large black-and-red book balanced on top of the drugs trolley, the Controlled Drugs book, enabling careful monitoring of any addictive drug such as morphine, which has to be signed in and out by two nurses, in case it is stolen. Addiction is common amongst nurses and doctors. There is no up-to-date or conclusive information regarding statistics, but a survey some time ago by Alcohol Concern and Drugscope, on the misuse of drugs and alcohol by NHS staff, suggested that 60 per cent of employers across all sectors had employees with alcohol problems, and 27 per cent with drug misuse. I can only imagine that figure has increased. Of course it's mostly low-level partying and drinking too much. A work hard, play harder mantra; a 999 night at the Ministry of Sound in Elephant and Castle, an example of frontline staff letting off steam; the regular club nights now organised by five medical schools, offering the chance to drink to excess with other frontline staff – and I'd imagine a good few of those medical students and nurses take drugs in the same way as, if not more than, any other young people in nightclubs.

But there is something deeper than that for NHS staff who have been in the job for many years. A GP I know regularly sees NHS staff who are battling addiction and depression. 'I try and see them once a week,' she says. 'The doctors particularly are a very high suicide risk. They're so highly stressed and have easy access to everything. And they don't attempt suicide. They do it.' Despite easy access to drugs, anaesthetic agents of sedation and paralysis, for example, I've known of a couple of doctors and nurses who have had serious addiction issues and who have ended up dying by suicide without those drugs, in dramatic and violent ways. There is now a twenty-four-hour helpline for doctors who need counselling, run by the General Medical Council. I don't know of any equivalent for nurses, though. There's often talk about the random drug-testing of doctors and nurses, but of course it's never been instigated – there would be no NHS.

I walk past the ward office and the large main area with six babies on life-support machines, with ventilators doing the work of the babies' underdeveloped lungs, and dozens of beeping noises and nurses bustling between them; then the SCBU nursery to my left, where the babies are not as sick, require less support and so have a higher baby-to-nurse ratio. The contrast between the two sides is immense, the walkway between them like a border separating two countries: NICU politically unsafe, and SCBU more stable and quieter. All of the babies on the NICU side are ventilated – that is, on life-support machines and intubated with breathing tubes, the endotracheal intubation first described by Hippocrates (460–375 BC).

NICU is noisy, despite the nurses' best efforts. Sensory overload has long been recognised as having a significant negative effect on a baby's future development, the sound and light exposure leading to sensory-processing problems and learning difficulties. Still, the NICU room is electric, bright with overhead lights, and noisy with the slamming of bins; the nurse having to think over the background buzzing of the oscillators, the sounds of suctioning and alarms. But the babies do not always startle: a testament to how sick they are. The fundamental reflexes that should be involuntary are absent. The nurses try and limit sound and noise by speaking in whispers, dimming the lights and placing towels over the tops of incubators at certain times of day. But this, too, may have a negative effect. Premature babies' auditory cortex is at a crucial stage of development: we need to hear language in order to learn it. But most of the environmental noise is white noise: chugging, banging, suctioning. These babies are fragile, on the edge of life, somewhere between worlds; they have immature lungs and a lack of surfactant – the substance that keeps the air sacs in the lungs open. They have yet to develop proper immune systems; their kidneys do not yet work properly and their gastrointestinal systems are fragile. The babies are at high risk of bleeding to the brain.

Neonatal nurses respond by being regimented. If babies thrive on and love routine and structure, then these nurses reflect that even more. You can tell, if you've worked around nurses for long enough, their speciality and which department they work in. Later in my career I spend a long time teaching multidisciplinary groups of nurses from all areas of the hospital, and it always surprises me that I can tell an A&E nurse from a scrub nurse, from a neonatal nurse. But I can. In a room full of nurses training in resuscitation, a friend and I run a poll to see if we can correctly guess where people work, based on where in the room they choose to sit. The nurses at the back looking terrified are scrub nurses: they are task-orientated and have little contact with patients; they have a high rate of failing the training and having to redo it. The nurses at the front are often intensive-care or A&E, ready to question the trainers, rather than the other way around. The nurse specialists sit at the sides and lean back in their chairs, looking bored. The latecomers, sadly, are healthcare assistants from medical wards and care of the elderly wards, or doctors who look annoyed at having to attend training with nurses and invariably ask to leave early, to attend to more important matters. There is always a nurse who sleeps during the training, to the extent that they are asked to stand in order to keep awake. Even then, sometimes they close their eyes while standing.

Neonatal nurses seemingly never get tired. They are often small and quick and fit. They flit from baby to baby and can multitask like nobody's business. Control and timing are everything. They are in charge and, regardless of how sick the babies are, it's the nurses leading the babies and not the other way round. They decide when the baby will have cares (eyes washed, mouth freshened), when the nappy needs changing, when the baby should be left alone from the doctors trying to cannulate them or the physios percussing their tiny chests as if they are miniature drums. Neonatal nurses would make excellent wedding planners. They organise and prioritise care in a grand way, with two or three babies to look after who require their breathing tubes suctioning or their ventilators weaned; physio-therapy or turning, observations, nasogastric feeding and drug administration. They need to piggyback the inotropes: replacing one syringe for another in tandem, carefully reducing the level of one strong heart drug and increasing the next, while all the time closely observing the baby's arterial blood pressure for swings. A mistake can lead to high blood pressure and the risk of the baby having a stroke. And there is no pattern. Each baby responds differently to the sensitive drugs, and the nurses, with their experience, simply get a feel for things.

Other times there are strict formulas, and neonatal nurses need to be good at mathematics, at preparing medication, working out doses. This need for competence at calculating mathematical formulas is not a new nursing task. The

Charaka-saṃhita is a Sanskrit text on Ayurveda (Indian trad-itional medicine) and one of the two foundational Hindu texts of this field that have survived from first-century-BC India. It advises that nurses 'must be knowledgeable, skilled at preparing formulations and dosage, sympathetic towards everyone and clean'.

A decimal point out of place, during a complex drug calcu-lation, can lead to the death of a baby. The symbol for nanograms and the symbol for micrograms look similar, yet they are a thousand times apart. My colleague once adminis-tered a thousand-times dose of a strong drug to a baby. The baby survived, but my friend – a junior nurse like me – died a little, over and over again. She carried the guilt like a cloak. I work with nurses who refuse to use calculators, as they don't trust them. They calculate in their heads all day, working out multiple complex sums in the loud, noisy and demanding environment of NICU. Calculations at 4 a.m. after being awake on twelve-and-a-half-hour night shifts, after five such nights without sleep:

The baby weighs 1.697 kg, has an IV of Dopamine 40 mg in 50 ml. What will the IV infusion rate be set at, to deliver 12.5 mcg/kg/min?

It terrifies me. I got a D in GCSE maths, and numbers move around my head with no anchor. I always check and check and recheck any calculations. I write endless lists. I'm impressed by my colleagues who, despite having a thousand jobs in their heads, can make sense of this, and time everything perfectly. Even so, it is a surprise to me when at 4 a.m. these meticulous nurses, who are almost obsessed with infection control and structure and priorities, shout loudly enough that I come running from the special-care area into the main intensive-care area. The nurses have laid out a long table, with white plastic tablecloths, upon which is a buffet: sausage rolls, cheese, sandwiches, juice, chicken legs, quiche, pizza and even vol-au-vents – it's like being in my nan's dining room at Christmas. Paper plates are piled up to one side and, if it wasn't for the babies in the room, the sound of the machines and the uniforms, you'd have thought you were at any family party or wedding reception. 'Ten minutes,' says the nurse in charge. And we all eat, chat, have a drink and then put everything in a black bin bag, wash our hands and get back to work. I am exhausted and the buffet is a welcome relief. I've been working extra shifts, long day after long day, in order to save enough to take a break and go backpacking around India. I am sharing a room in the nurses' accommodation in a bid to save money, with a friend who works the opposite nights to my days. We never see each other. She is working when I am sleeping, and vice versa, so we can split the already-cheap rent. The short break and the food help me to stay awake.

Later, at the end of our shift, one of the agency nurses walks with me to the lifts. I ask about the buffet and she explains that it happens every day, regardless. Sometimes the doctors bring in doughnuts, too. And the nurses take it in turns to bring snacks.

'It's so great working here. Those ten minutes of looking after ourselves – the nurses – do the babies no harm. In fact it helps them. We're all fed and watered, and we feel looked-after ourselves. Of course it's probably breaking every hospital rule...'

The staffroom is next to the sluice, the place where dirty clinical waste is chucked down a chute, almost like a toilet. And where once, after a baby had died, she was put in a basket, then placed in the sluice room to wait for the porters who would come and take her to the mortuary. After some time of seemingly being dead, the baby girl began to cry. Her parents were in the office, with a note on the door that said 'Confidential Meeting in Progress', sitting on stained sofas and crying into scratchy tissues. The doctor next to me was telling them that their daughter was simply too early, and her life couldn't be maintained, until we heard a knock on the door from the junior sister, who had gone into the sluice to investigate the crying; she poked her head around the door and, in a serious tone, said, 'A word, please. An urgent word.' The baby lived for a short while only, but the parents had the shock of experiencing grief twice. 'We made a mistake,' the doctor told them, 'and there is no easy way to tell you.' They named her Hope.

You can sometimes smell melaena from the sluice – a foul kind of blood-filled diarrhoea that suggests a baby's abdominal bleed – while you are trying to eat a sandwich. But today the staffroom smells only of coffee and sweat, and of the pickled-onion Monster Munch snacks that one of the nurses is eating for breakfast. There's nowhere to sit, so I perch next to Barbara, the kind of nurse who can stop a baby crying from across a room. After the handover I walk to my bed space.

Baby Emmanuel is wrapped up like a tiny precious gift, but instead of being in wrapping paper, he is inside a supermarket sandwich bag, which acts like a mini-greenhouse. He was born much too early: at twenty-four weeks, the legal cut-off age for an abortion in the UK. Preterm birth, which happens before thirty-seven weeks pregnant, is the largest cause of newborn deaths, and the second-biggest cause of deaths in children under five. Globally, one in ten pregnancies will result in premature birth, and this number is rising. People are having babies later in life, and multiple births as a result of IVF. Emmanuel's head is unnaturally big, his eyes wide as he blinks slowly. A small, thin feeding tube snakes into his nose, held down with a piece of tape: he's too little to suck. His skin is ashen, with blue-grey veins patterning his scalp. He looks pretty cosy, though, wrapped up and inside a see-through incubator. But everything fights against him. He had a rocky start: as well as being born much too early, he was even smaller than expected, weighing just 900 grams, and suffered a bleed into his brain.

The first thing I do when I reach Emmanuel's bed space is check the oxygen and suction attached to the wall. Today the tubing is pushed in correctly and, as I switch on the wall suction, I test it on my gloved hand to check the pressures, glance at the correct-sized suction catheters in a long holder, and make sure the oxygen is set at the right level and working, and that there is a bag valve mask with a correct-sized mask attached nearby, in case the baby's endotracheal tube falls out. There are a million things that can go wrong and seemingly minor checks that – if not done correctly – have life-threatening possibilities. If the oxygen is set too low, or too high, the baby can develop retinopathy of prematurity, among other complications, and blindness can occur. If the baby's oxygen saturation levels swing (these babies get nicknamed 'swingers'), other complications can happen and can lead to multiple devastating injuries. If the suction is not available and the baby's tube gets blocked, the baby can suffocate to death; or if the bag valve mask is not available, the baby becomes hypoxic and can end up brain-damaged, or with intestinal ischaemia, or bradycardic (low heart rate); if the wrong-sized mask is fitted onto the bag and pressed on the baby's face, slightly too large, it can hit the vagal nerve and cause life-threatening bradycardia.

Mistakes happen everywhere and occur increasingly in the NHS. 'Never events' – serious clinical medical mistakes – are now at their highest in four years. These incidents, which are entirely preventable, have the potential to cause a patient harm or even death.

After ensuring that the emergency equipment is working and correct, I check Emmanuel, a quick assessment: **ABCDE**.

Airway: Check the tube placement, make sure Emmanuel's airway is not at risk.

Breathing: Check his oxygen levels, listen to his chest, look for symmetry, percuss his chest to check it is resonant (normal), hyper-resonant or dull (indicating a serious problem).

Circulation: Listen to his heart, check his arterial blood pressure, feel his skin temperature, press his foot and let go and see how long the colour takes to return, then do the same on his sternum.

Disability: Look at his tone, his posture, his fontanelle, his pupil reaction and his conscious level.

Exposure: Examine his body for anything else: swelling, bleeds, marks, bruises, front and back, top to toe.

This is the way nurses and doctors worldwide assess all critically ill patients, whether the patient is one or one hundred. But a baby's anatomy is different, and each clue is important for an assessing nurse. Babies (and children to a lesser degree) compensate to ensure they protect their vital organs for as long as possible. Babies keep their blood pressure at normal levels, for example, until they are about to have a cardiac arrest, whereas 80 per cent of adults show clinical signs of deterioration for twenty-four hours before arresting. This means that nurses looking after children, and especially babies, have to be eagle eyed. Some of the physiological signs that babies show when deteriorating are anatomical: their ribs, for example, sit vertically, so they are unable to take deep breaths, and instead take faster breaths, using accessory muscles to suck in air wherever possible, even bobbing their heads and flaring their nostrils. But there are advanced compensatory mechanisms that cannot be fully explained by anatomy. A baby in serious respiratory failure will grunt, blowing out air in such a way that they are forcing their own alveolar in the lungs open in the same way as a mechanical ventilator, making their own PEEP (positive end expiratory pressure), which is one of the settings the doctors prescribe on their complicated life-support machines. By keeping the smallest parts of their lungs open in this way, they are avoiding having to blow the difficult first part – like a child at a birthday party asking a parent to start blowing the balloon. Only babies have this ability to grunt, to compensate. They keep their blood pressure normal to perfuse (send oxygenated blood to) their brains much longer than an adult can. They have spots on the top of the head – the fontanelle – allowing brain swelling that would certainly kill an adult. They have soft, pliable bones that are difficult to break. In many ways they are so fragile, but their instincts are incredibly strong. An adult loses these protective abilities, or perhaps the will to survive at all costs. As we become physically stronger, life makes us more emotionally fragile.

Emmanuel's mum, Joy, a smiling Ugandan woman, sits next to his incubator with a giant breast in her hand, pumping the milk that will eventually drip into his tube. She chats away. First about Uganda, where she says the people are kind and the politics are complicated. Then about what her son will be. 'His dad is six foot four,' she says, 'so he'll probably be a basketball player or something. Though I'm the academic one. My granddad was a doctor. My dad a doctor. I studied law, spent most of my career working with asylum-seekers.'

She's a humble woman, self-deprecating and embarrassed when I remark that she must have helped so many people.

'You can't imagine the horrors they run from,' she says.

I smile at her every now and then, while busy organising a long list of drugs for her son. He's having regular caffeine into a nasogastric tube, to ensure that he remembers to breathe. Caffeine is a central respiratory stimulant and is widely used for small babies who suffer from apnoea (periods of prolonged breath-holding). 'Like me in the mornings,' Joy says, when I explain to her what it is. But there's concern in her voice: I hear a change over the swooshing of the breast pump, the sound of the monitors alarming, the slamming of the yellow clinical waste bins, the shoes on the overpolished floor.

'Do you want to pick him up? Give him a cuddle?'

She looks at me with sudden tears appearing at the corners of her eyes. 'Will it hurt him? I'm afraid.'

'Of course not. It will help him. Nothing better than a cuddle.'

I know that Joy has not yet held her son. We discussed it during handover. The nurses are worried that she has not bonded yet. Nurses understand that as well as surgical and technological interventions, family-centred care can have a significant impact on a baby's cognitive outcomes. Emmanuel will not, I predict, be a basketball player or a medical doctor or a human-rights lawyer. And I imagine Joy knows that. His heart has already stopped a number of times in the ten days since he was born. His bowel is not working properly. He will be lucky to reach his milestones. He could be deaf or blind, and have significant learning disabilities, as well as physical health problems. He might need a lifetime of care.

With Joy beside him, Emmanuel is somehow improving, clinging to life. It's tricky to get him out of the incubator, and there's a level of risk involved. The breathing tube can easily become dislodged. It hasn't been long since we've stopped the cruel practice of stitching a tube onto a baby's mouth to hold it in position without using anaesthetic: there was a medically-led belief that premature babies did not experience pain. Thankfully, Emmanuel's tube is held in place with white tape. Despite the tape, I worry about the risk of his breathing tube falling out, if I move him. But the risks to him, if Joy doesn't have the opportunity to hold her son, are far greater. And Joy's mental health is at stake, too. Studies have found that women are twice as likely to suffer postnatal depression when a baby is born prematurely than at full term. Childbirth is like a soul splitting in two: that's why it hurts so much. In not holding him, Joy is still missing a half of herself. He is not real, not whole, until she holds him. And nor is she.

With care, taking many minutes to do so, I untangle Emmanuel from his bed of wires and place him in Joy's hands. He looks even smaller outside the incubator, but he does not cry. He looks at his mum for the longest time without blinking, and she looks back at him, and in a few short minutes they fall in love.

'He's perfect,' she says.

I agree, looking up and smiling at my colleague, who is standing with her hand on her heart. Everything is against him, but in this moment I remember that everything is possible. Isaac Newton – like Emmanuel – was born prematurely and was not expected to live more than a few hours. It is something special to watch a mother on NICU. The miracle of a baby seems somehow even more miraculous. Joy looks at Emmanuel. He is full of possibilities.

'He's going to be okay, isn't he? I just know it.'

'You both are,' I reply.

I'm in the Special-Care Baby Unit on my own today, as it's so busy, and with four babies to care for. I like it in here most of the time. The babies are almost universally adorable and are getting better, likely to go home. There is a calm from the parents, a belief and hope that their child is moving from the edge of life to solid ground. The entire unit can, however, face bed crises, and it's not unusual in busy winters when there is an increase in the number of patients throughout the hospital, due to infectious diseases – respiratory infections mainly – to have an extra baby in a basin, in what we call the 'sink space' underneath the sink. We half-open the taps at those times, to prevent the baby getting splashed. There are strict protective guidelines on the architectural structure of neonatal units, and on the amount of space for chairs around each bed, to facilitate bonding between baby and parents, though hospitals have times when they're bursting at the seams and some days it is simply a case of needs must.

But today it's warm and quiet, and the babies are not as sick as the intensive-care babies next door. There are no mums here at the moment, which is unusual. The nurses do everything they can to keep mother and baby as one unit. It is quite different in private hospitals. In maternity units in some private hospitals, babies are taken from the mum shortly after birth to be cared for in the nursery, by a very capable stranger. But still a stranger. There's a postcard on the lockers in the staff changing room in the hospital here that says: 'Show me the child at seven, and I'll show you the man', and one of the nurses has written underneath it: 'Show me the baby and the mother at twelve hours, and I'll show you the man.'

David's mum, Mandy, is a sex worker from Lambeth, who has had nine children already, all taken into care. David is the quietest baby in SCBU. He doesn't move much. He is quite different from the demographic of other babies I've cared for who are born to drug-addicted mothers, who can be twitching or suffering seizures. He is wearing a knitted blue hat and has a machine called CPAP delivering air via two tiny prongs sitting just inside his nostrils. His nappy, although the smallest nappy in production, still swamps him, and his twig-like legs triangle out of the sides; his skin is the skin of old people, loose and wrinkly, hanging off his bones like an ill-fitting outfit. He has long feet and long fingers – the kind of thing we comment on to parents, in a bid to normalise the situation, move Mandy's eyes away from the medical equipment puncturing his skin. 'Look at his fingers – piano-player fingers.'

David's face, although partially hidden by the prongs and by a nasogastric tube in his nostril and taped to his cheek and around his ear, is quite beautiful, his eyes are open wide and framed by long, curled eyelashes. It is a cruel truth that the most beautiful babies are the sickest, or have the worst chance at life. But it is a truth. David's eyes are covered today with an eye-mask, much like the one I wear on sunny mornings at home in bed. He has jaundice and the whites of his eyes (sclera) are yellow. This is not uncommon; 85 per cent of preterm babies have clinically apparent jaundice, and need photo-therapy and regular blood tests to monitor their liver function. The *Huangdi Neijing*, an ancient text that has been the core writing on Chinese medicine for more than two millennia, describes the liver as the general of an army. In Chinese medi-cine, the liver houses *hun*, the ethereal soul or cloud soul. It is with sun that we treat liver jaundice in the West. David is naked, apart from the eye-mask and nappy, and is lying underneath a sun lamp, a miniature person sunbathing. The fluorescent lamp above him rains strobe nightclub lighting, providing photo-oxidation that adds oxygen to the bilirubin – the substance made during the breakdown of red blood cells – so that it dissolves easily in water. This makes it easier for a baby's liver to break down and remove the large amounts of bilirubin that indicate jaundice in their blood. David looks pretty relaxed in the neon light, like a hand in a shellac nail-salon light-box.

I read David's notes, work out the timings of his medi-cation, look at the patterns of his observations, his care plan. There is very little information about his mum, and none about his dad. There is a suspicion that he has been prenatally exposed to crack cocaine, as well as cigarettes and alcohol, and Mandy did not attend any antenatal appointments. Her diet, I can assume, contained no vitamins or nutrients, and folic acid was out of the question. David was born early and small, yet despite his inauspicious start, he appears medically robust. He doesn't show any signs yet of foetal alcohol syndrome, although he might have it. Foetal alcohol spectrum disorder (FASD) is of unknown prevalence in the UK, and any prenatal exposure to alcohol is a risk factor. There is no treatment, and the damage to the child's brain and organs cannot be reversed. It is suggested that children with FASD often get misdiagnosed with conditions such as autism and ADHD. When alcohol passes from the mother into the foetus's body, the baby lacks oxygen and the nutrients needed for its brain and organs to grow properly. David's future is full of uncertainties. Everything is against him. The general of his army might be treatable on SCBU with phototherapy, but the general of his mother's army – her own liver, a commander of chaos – is a war living on in David.

The function of nursing is similar to the function of the liver, which is in charge of infection control, of wound care – making enzymes and proteins involved in blood clotting and tissue repair – and of nutrition, digesting food to retain goodness. Nurses can't eliminate toxins as the liver does, but we certainly spend a lot of time trying to change the focus of bad things by introducing hope, comfort and kindness.

Grainne relieves me for a break. She's a neonatal advanced practitioner nurse and does a lot of teaching about ethical responsibility, as well as the physiology of preterm babies. She is excellent with equipment, too. Any issues with ventilators, setting up complicated tubing or even the blood-gas-analysis machine, Grainne is always able to fix it. She is obsessed with applied physics, and has tried many times to explain the complicated formulas about dynamic and static compliance in relation to pressure changes, and the like. She never gets exasperated with me when I ask her to re-explain, in the simplest language possible. Understanding physics, although it is an important part of nursing, has never been my strong suit.

'Poor little lamb. I'd like to take him home, wouldn't you?'

We peer at David's face, lift his eye-mask, smile at his curled eyelashes.

'What's the story? Will his mum come in at all?'

She shakes her head. 'Never does. I've looked after a few of the others. The last one died. A couple have been adopted, a few are in long-term foster care.'

'Why does she keep getting pregnant? Surely it must be traumatic. Why does she not have long-term contraception?'

Grainne shakes her head again. 'I know. What's his life going to be like?'

Mandy does come in, though. She is unable to stand still, a mess of sores on her arms and unwashed hair, talking at a hundred miles an hour. She smells of alcohol and sweat.

'How is he? Is he getting better? Will he be okay? I'm going to wash my hands, but I won't wake him up.' She scratches her arms as she talks.

'Hi.' I smile, telling myself not to judge her, and introduce myself. 'He's doing well. David's robust.'

There is a child-protection order on him already, but supervised contact is allowed. I make a risk assessment of Mandy. Is she too out of it? Is she likely to grab him and try and run off? I watch her face watching David's face, her frown whenever the CPAP machine beeps.

I nod and she walks to the sink in the corner of the room. She takes a long, long time washing her hands, I notice, and then she dries them and begins washing them again. 'I'm pretty sure they're the cleanest hands in the hospital,' I say.

'Well, I don't want to give him any germs. Not that I'll wake him up, but some germs travel anyway.'

When she sits down, I see two wet patches where Mandy's milk has soaked through her T-shirt. I hand her some tissues, but she shrugs. 'My body knows my baby,' she says. 'I've had nine already.' David is being fed breast milk donated by another mother. Wet nursing, where the nursing name originates, is alive and well today, and the idea of it is still at the heart of nursing. Helping someone who needs help.

The room is very quiet, very hot. I need to start doing the nasogastric feed for the baby in the next cot, dripping her mum's breast milk slowly through a 20 ml syringe (sometimes taping it to the side of the bassinet with sticking plaster, if the babies all need a feed at the same time, as it drips so slowly into their tiny tubes).

But I pull a plastic chair up next to Mandy instead. I doubt she gets to talk to many people. I don't imagine she has friends, or family, or support. She doesn't engage with social services, and Grainne said she is in and out of a relationship with an abusive and controlling man. He might be the father of David; maybe not.

'Ten babies,' I say. 'I'm not sure I could go through child-birth ten times.'

She looks at David, then up at me. Her own eyes have yellow edges. 'Did they tell you that I don't keep them. My babies. All adopted or in care.'

I nod. 'It's in your notes. Must be hard.'

'I'd be a really good mum,' she says. 'But they won't let me try. They keep telling me to go on the pill or be sterilised. Can you believe that? Like the Nazis? But I think it's different now. I can keep David. I've got a place to live and everything's more sorted out.'

Mandy doesn't seem to have any capacity to imagine the harm she is causing her children. She doesn't discuss what life will be like for them. She talks for a long time about her feelings and how she might be able to get her children back, how the social workers were too quick to judge and nobody gave her a chance. But it is impossible to resent her. Mandy does not want the life she leads, she did not choose it. We don't talk about her own childhood; we don't need to.

'I feel so empty without my babies, but I won't have any more,' she says. 'I just want to keep David. He's my heart and soul. I'll miss being pregnant, though. I love being pregnant. Especially when they start to move. That feeling that something is alive inside you, with a heartbeat. It makes me feel alive.'

In the next bed space is Sophia. She was born with spina bifida, a serious type of the condition that caused a mye-lomeningocele, whereby her spine and its protective layer have pushed outside her body. This is associated with serious infections and significant damage to the spinal cord. I change her very carefully, remembering the time I had to change the nappies and Babygros of conjoined twins, as a student nurse. A simple thing, and yet it was tricky and my hands were shaking. I feared I'd hurt them somehow, simply by getting them caught in poppers or Velcro. They were stuck together at the abdomen, curled around each other, both looking at me. Tiny speech marks. The mentor nurse who had asked me to change them said it was good practice for me. I remember telling her I'd never changed such anatomically complicated babies and, even though it was only their nappies and Baby-gros, it took me half an hour. She shook her head. 'That's not what I meant,' she said.

Sophia's parents – Emma and Helen – spend long hours every day holding her impossibly small hand through a hole in the side of the incubator, watching her face, singing to her, trying not to look at her insides spilling out. They did everything right: folic acid, outpatient appointments, NCT classes; they read every book and prepared the most beautiful nursery for her. Emma shows me a photograph of it. 'We went to town. A friend of mine is an artist, so we had her do a painting. See the butterflies? We knew she'd be a girl. I'm so happy she is! She's already got a more extensive wardrobe than me! Imagine.'

Sophia's future – like David's – is full of uncertainties. She may not walk. She might be incontinent. Almost certainly Sophia will suffer a life that is medicalised, and full of hospitals and hurdles.

I take Sophia to theatre, where everything is waiting: the first hurdle of her life. Her parents hold hands on the way; Emma, still recovering from the birth, is in a wheelchair that I'm pushing, while the porter has Sophia's incubator. Helen walks beside us, holding Emma's hand. I notice how tightly they hold on to each other: their knuckles turn white.

6

Somewhere Under My Left Ribs

I took a deep breath and listened to the old brag of my heart.
I am, I am, I am.

Sylvia Plath, *The Bell Jar*

The landscape of theatres must be terrifying for patients, but it's becoming normal for me. It's amazing what you can get used to. Life wasn't always like this.

The first operation that I watch is a heart-lung transplant. I am nineteen years old and still a student nurse. The operation takes so long: over twelve hours. It requires a team of surgeons to behave like a relay team; but instead of a baton, they pass between them a human heart and lungs. I've been looking after the patient waiting for the new set of lungs that day: a fourteen-year-old boy named Aaron suffering from cystic fibrosis, who is confined to bed, oxygen tubes inserted into his nose, with a tired, wet cough and sallow grey skin. I help him get ready for the operation. I rub cocoa butter onto his dry knees, take away his Game Boy and swear to guard it with my life. I wet his lips with a small salmon-pink sponge that I dip in sterile water, not wanting to risk the tiniest possibility of him being exposed to any germs.

Aaron's room glows with lights in the shape of stars and moons surrounding his hospital bed and a journal is hidden under his pillow. There is a small corkboard next to his bed that his stepdad has Blu-tacked to the wall, covered in a mosaic of photographs of him with his friends, every single one of them smiling. It is a common thing for a child's hospital room to be personalised. Aside from the oxygen piped through the wall and the suction canister with its thick transparent tubing, it could be a typical teenage bedroom.

We chat almost as if nothing is happening, but when the porters come to help me transfer Aaron to the anaesthetic room, he grabs his mum. 'Don't go before I'm asleep,' he says. He looks at me. 'And you will be there the whole time?'

'I'll be there. You ready?'

He shakes his head no. I nod to the porters anyway and they begin pushing his bed through the doors, out of the ward and down the corridor. One of the porters, a cheerful young woman, whistles continuously. The walls are young-child-friendly and are painted with animals and flowers. Children walk past us pushing drip-stands, their parents or a nurse smiling behind them. The porter whistles; Aaron shakes his head again. His mum holds his hand, walking quickly beside the bed. I have one eye on the monitor at the end of Aaron's bed, which measures the oxygen in his blood. I will it not to drop. 'Not now,' I say in my head. 'Steady, steady.' I've heard stories of children getting worse in broken-down lifts, oxygen running out and full cardiac arrests being badly managed, until a lift engineer is found. I am anxious, but have already learned the face that nurses know best. I slow my own breathing and movements and focus on portraying an easy-going body language and a soft smile. One of our nursing lecturers, when explaining the benefit of our clinical placements in gaining experience, told us that if the patient ever sees an experienced nurse looking worried, it means they are likely dead already.

Theatre is a maze of corridors and trolleys, covered in sterile blue sheets, containing internal defibrillator paddles and difficult airway kits. The theatre nurses walk so quickly, their clogs squeaking quietly on the shining floor, their half-done-up theatre cloaks billowing out behind them as if they are magicians. There are numerous equipment rooms; in one the nurse kneeling down with her checklist, which she signs off every morning and every night: expiry date, number of sets, date of new batch ordered. There is an autoclave machine in the corner where some equipment is being sterilised; the arterial blood-gas machine that tells the nurse how well the anaesthetist is getting on, and whether the patient is being oxygenated or is full of carbon-dioxide gases. The air in the winding, low-lit corridors seems to be thick, holding onto memory like a smell. It tells stories, if you listen hard enough, of the wrong kidney being removed, or the time when the electricity stopped and the generator did not kick in; or the occasion when the patient was defibrillated and the oxygen was not removed, and there was an explosion that sounded like a bomb going off and resulted in the anaesthetic nurse receiving a nasty head injury and admission to intensive care. If walls could talk.

Many of us pass through the operating theatre largely without memory. We go to sleep and wake up, without examining too closely what happened in between. Theatre nurses see everything. Sometimes funny things: the surgeon and nurse found in the linen cupboard in a state of undress. The men having minor operations who get erections, due to the anaesthetic, and a penis that goes up and down with each movement of the surgeon's blade, often in time with the music. I work with a surgeon much later on whose scrub trousers fall down during a crucial moment and who happens to be wearing Bart Simpson underwear; a nurse awkwardly attempts to pull them up, while he shouts, 'Leave them, leave them alone!'

But theatre is also the place where life and death are literally in someone else's hands. Most of the time everything goes right, but when it goes wrong it is a disaster. The organised, calm, sterile environment can look like a war zone when a patient suddenly deteriorates. Anaesthesiologists do their best to predict which patient groups will be problematic – the obese, smokers, pregnant women, and such – though there are always surprises. There are patients who claim they were awake during the operation and unable to move, a phenomenon explained by the paralysis agent given to them and their lack of reaction to the accompanying sedative. There are patients who react badly to anaesthetic drugs and have a dangerous drop in blood pressure, an occasional cardiac arrest.

I have looked after such patients, who are told post-operatively that things were a little unstable in theatre, but the surgeon managed to stabilise them. The language of nursing is sometimes difficult. A heart cell beats in a Petri dish. A single cell. And another person's heart cell in a Petri dish beats in a different time. Yet if the two touch, they beat in unison. A doctor can explain this with science. But a nurse knows that the language of science is not enough. The nurse in theatre translates 'your husband / wife / child died three times in there, but today was a good day and, with a large amount of electricity and some chest compressions that probably broke a few ribs, we managed to get them back' into something that we can hear. A strange sort of poetry.

I try not to think of what can happen in theatre, of all that can – and has – gone wrong. I adopt my relaxed-on-the-outside, panicking-on-the-inside pose until we arrive in the anaesthetic room, which is full of reassuring equipment and a very relaxed-looking and smiling anaesthetist. 'Okay then, Mum. Hi, Aaron.' The anaesthetist introduces herself and keeps eye contact with Aaron, while all the time the operating-department assistant buzzes around in the background, preparing the monitoring and labelling syringes. I stand at the end of the bed, near enough to reach out and pull Aaron's mum away, if necessary, in the seconds after Aaron has fallen asleep from the gas and air and before she needs to be ushered out. We do not want her to witness the next stage, after a patient is put to sleep: eyes taped shut, head tipped back as far as possible and a tube pushed into his trachea, needles passed into veins, remaining clothing removed. Skin is then painted a muddy copper with Betadine iodine solution until a patient no longer looks human, more like a piece of meat. Ready for the surgeons, of whom in 1800 Lord Thurlow, a Member of Parliament, stated, 'There is no more science in surgery than in butchering.' Surgery was considered such a lowly profession that even women were admitted during the Middle Ages, until the 1700s, when surgical training moved into the universities, from which women were barred. Attitudes towards, and public perception of, surgery have moved on a lot more than that of nursing, which at times seems to be heading in the opposite direction.

I am waiting, with my teeth pressed together, for the awful moment between a child being anaesthetised and a parent having to kiss them goodbye and leave them in the hands of strangers. I feel in awe of the anaesthetist, who is cool and calm and reassuring, despite having sole charge of a complicated and high-risk patient.

The next time I go to theatre I will watch an operation with a fellow nursing student: Jess. I'll be impressed with the anaesthetist then, too, in awe of him, until Jess tells me she's had an affair with him. She will lift her surgical mask up higher and higher during the operation, until I can barely even see her eyes. 'What are you doing?' I ask her. 'I've slept with everyone in here,' she says. 'Except the patient.'

Now I walk with Aaron's mum for a few moments outside the theatre, hug her, wish I could say something to help, search inside myself for comforting words.

'That was the worst moment of my life,' she says. 'The worst.'

I swear I'll never underestimate how hard it must be to entrust your child's life to strangers, no matter how expert they are.

Nurses can be found in the theatre corridors of all hospitals with their arms around a relative, reassuring them – or not – that the operation is going well. After we leave the stark white theatre corridors, I walk with Aaron's mum back to the ward, where she begins to cry. I sit with her for a while, without speaking. Eventually she looks at the clock.

'It will be hours and hours,' I say. 'All day. You need to fill the time. I'll head back shortly, to be with Aaron.'

'I'm meeting my sister,' she says. 'I'll try to keep busy.'

I smile at her. I do not tell her what she wants to hear. I have learned that already. The previous week, one of the first babies I'd looked after was going for a relatively straightforward operation to fix a hole in his heart. 'He'll be fine,' I said repeatedly to his parents. But he was not fine. He did not come back from theatre. He died on the operating table. I got it very wrong. His parents were distraught and confused. I told the nurse in charge my mistake, and I cried and cried. 'They won't even remember what you told them,' she said. 'It wouldn't make any difference. You did nothing wrong.' But I know that my words were wrong. I can still see his yellow cardigan.

I don't tell Aaron's mum that Aaron will be fine. I'd never tell any relative that: I've learned my lesson. Because none of us really knows.

'Try and keep busy,' I say. 'Time will move very slowly.'

Time is a funny thing. If we are waiting for a relative having an operation, it slows down, until each second becomes a minute, each minute an hour. Yet if we are a patient having an operation, time becomes shorter: we count down from ten, and there is nothing.

The large operating theatre is full of people, yet you could hear a pin drop. There is a radio on a shelf high up behind the surgeon's head, although it is silent. The reassuring sound of music when the operation is going well is absent. The words 'Turn the music down' in theatre mean that things are not going well – an artery has been nicked, there is a bleed, a drop in blood pressure or a cardiac arrest. But today the lack of music is simply reflective of the enormity of the situation. I am standing on a viewing tower with a clutch of medical students and junior doctors: a large operating theatre full of people is standard for interesting or groundbreaking cases, and teaching is common practice during operations. Nowadays operations are filmed and streamed to surgeons around the world, for teaching purposes and for advice from other doctors from various countries: the expert in the details of the procedure, who is based in LA, never needs to leave LA any more. There are screens displaying everything, but primarily for the people inside the room, and some distance away from the actual surgery. Most faces are studying the screens, watching the hands of the surgeon inside the patient, twisting and turning like a dancer's hands, moving skilfully around the beating heart in perfect synchronicity. I think I've never seen anything as beautiful as Aaron's heart beating in front of my eyes. Of course I see something even more beautiful, some years later, when I watch the tiniest flickering of my own baby's heart on an ultrasound screen.

Aaron is at the centre of the room. His body is by now a dugout canoe. The surgeon's hands are inside him. What a strange privilege to place your hands inside a human being, to touch a heart with your fingertips, to become briefly one. I think about that while watching the surgery: how the surgeon and the patient are one, like a mother and her unborn child, sharing the same shell of a body for a time. The room smells of chlorine, bleach and sweat. There is also a strange sharp, biting metallic smell, which might be blood. The walls are clean, but I know that the ECMO machine – the machine that carries the entirety of a person's circulating blood volume during some operations – once split open, and the walls and ceiling, and staff and equipment, were soaked with blood. A horror film.

I shudder and focus on a strand of Aaron's hair. It reminds me that he is not a carcass being butchered, but a boy obsessed with astronomy, whose battered Game Boy I have locked safely away. The surgeon's body is completely still above Aaron, his arms and hands the only part of him moving. The other surgeons around the table (I count four in total) are facing him, one of whom has a suction catheter, hoovering up blood around the surgeon's hands in order that he gets a better view. Another surgeon simply points a large overhead light inside Aaron. There are lights everywhere and it is ridiculously hot, even wearing thin scrubs. But there is never enough light. I look at all the surgery team – most of them men with grey hair, and the occasional woman – and imagine where in his medical career the light-holder is: how you progress from holding the light to suctioning blood, to dancing hands. It must take a lifetime of watching. I am fascinated with surgery, particularly at this tertiary-care teaching hospital where nothing is routine or, if it is, is performed on a child with complex and significant medical needs.

But today it isn't the surgeon that I am here to watch. Standing next to him a wide-shouldered woman, with thinning hair noticeable at the front of her cap, has her double-gloved hands in front of her body, her fingers starfished, palms down. Below her is a long table of metal instruments, shining diamonds on the stark white ceiling. Every so often the lead surgeon, or one of the assisting surgeons, will say something without lifting their eyes and then she picks up a metal instrument – a scalpel, a stitch, a pair of clamps or arterial forceps – and passes it to them, placing the handle in their hand in the way that you would pass scissors. Sometimes she passes things before the surgeon asks. A look burns between them. She is the scrub nurse. When an instrument is finished with, the scrub nurse turns her head and flicks her eyes to the nurse standing behind her, armed with a plastic tray, who then places that on a table behind the operating table. Nothing is removed from the room. Everything is counted, and counted again. 'In case the surgeon accidentally leaves a swab inside a cavity, a scalpel in a lung, a piece of gauze in intestines,' the scrub nurse tells me the following day in her gravelly voice. 'But we've lost worse. And if things are not going well, my instruments can get thrown and then lost.'

'Thrown?'

'By the surgeon. Occasionally even at the nurses.' She looks at me and narrows her eyes and smiles. 'It's a very stressful job.'

I have no idea if she is telling the truth, or even if she means the surgeon's job or hers is stressful, but I am too terrified to ask.

She has something sparky in her eyes that you can only see when close to her. I missed it before. There is a tiny hole on the side of her nose from a nose-ring, and I learn later that she is obsessed with motorbikes. She looks nothing like I imagine a nurse to look. I already know enough to realise that scrub nursing is not for me. Theatre nursing has now moved on to mean that nurses work across different areas, including the surgical admissions lounge, main theatres, recovery and day surgery, but at this time scrub nurses remain scrub nurses for a whole career, in the same way that night nurses could simply work nights for ever. Now all nurses work days and nights on rotation. I know that I'm not particularly organised, or good at standing still for hours, and the heat of the operating theatres is almost too much to bear. But I watch the heavy hands of that scrub nurse for hours during the operation. The way they are perfectly still, then suddenly purposeful, almost aggressive; then still once more, moving completely differently from the beautiful, delicate hands of the surgeon.

I watch the nurse's eyes. Imagine all she has seen. Her gaze rests occasionally on the surgery we've all come to witness, but then flies around the room, landing on the monitors behind the surgeon, where I see her eyes recording the vital signs; then on the perfusionist (the blood-machine expert) who is wearing a multicoloured bandana, sitting on a stool next to the cardiac-bypass machine, writing frantically on a clipboard. The bypass machine looks futuristic, twisting and turning tubes in a pattern, much like a complicated water-slide at a funfair. The nurse turns her head a fraction and glances at the assistant nurses by the door, at the organ-donation coordinator nurse, holding the box containing another person's heart and lungs. It is a plain square white box, with the words 'Human tissue' written on it. The scrub nurse's eyes rest on the box for a long time. Then she looks up at the organ-donation coordinator. Something passes between the two. Something that, at the time, I do not quite understand. But I appreciate the importance of what is happening. The room is alive with miracles: of technology, surgical technique, science and luck, alongside the sadness and loss that are recognised by the nurses.

The organ-donation coordinator is the person standing centre-court between life and death. Talking to families about donating the organs of a recently deceased loved one, in order that another can live. That Aaron can live. Over the years I listen to many organ-donation coordinators – all of them nurses from various backgrounds specialising in cardiac transplantation, living donors, or all roles related to different types of organ donation. They coordinate the time process between donor and recipient: a twenty-four-hour period during which the call can come at any time. Still, three people die in the UK every day while waiting for an organ. It should be compulsory, unless a person refuses. Opt out, not opt in – like it is in other countries. If a person would accept an organ if they were dying, then they should register as an organ donor themselves. Who would rather die than accept an organ? Nobody should die waiting for a kidney that is buried in the ground, disintegrating.

The heart can beat for seventy-two hours after a person is pronounced brain-dead. The organ-donation coordinator will discuss this with the donor's family, and try and help them understand that their loved one has died, despite the heart continuing to beat. The nurse will support them if they choose not to donate, or if they want the heart to stop beating completely, after which time it is still possible to donate heart valves. Someone who donates organs might help numerous people: one kidney to a person on dialysis in Southampton, the other kidney to a child in renal failure in Bradford; the liver to a recovering alcoholic in Dumfries; bone, tendons, cartilage, skin, corneas, a pancreas, lungs, heart – all split and delivered to patients who are desperate, and some of whom will die on the waiting list unless they receive a transplant. What greater gift is there than that? There are people, too, who donate a kidney while they are alive, well and simply want to save another life. A level of kindness that I can't imagine.

It is unusual to see the organ-donation coordinator at the recipient's end. The medical courier usually delivers the organs after they are put in a bag with a nutrient-rich fluid – which looks like a half-melted Slush Puppie. When a family consents to organ donation (or in the case of many countries, the patient has consented before death), there is a period of time before anything happens: time for tests and goodbyes. The organ-donation coordinator will do everything in her power to make this time less stressful for the family. Organ-donation coordinators in America, for example, sometimes make moulds of patient's hands, and even bring in the family's pets. The organ-donation coordinator then stays with the donor, caring for the patient after death, being with their family, as they are hollowed out into a shell of bones – parts of them returning to live in another person's shell.

I stand until I can no longer feel my toes, and the teams – including the scrub nurse – have changed three times. So many long hours. Despite being the most tired I've ever felt, I have never felt more awake. My eyes are wide open.

It is a matter of a few weeks since the operation and Aaron looks like a totally different child. His skin is brighter, the oxygen tubes have vanished and the wet, hacking cough is completely gone. His bedroom is a mess of books and games and cards.

'I love strawberry ice-cream,' he says. 'I never liked it before but now I could eat it all day. Breakfast, lunch and dinner. And snacks.' Aaron looks at me meaningfully. He is convinced that somehow he has taken on personality characteristics and emotions from his donor. It is the lungs that Aaron needed to treat his cystic fibrosis, though it is the attached heart that he thinks about most.

He is not alone in his belief that the heart houses more than muscle, cells and valves. Professor Bruce Hood, a cognitive neuroscientist at the University of Bristol, tested information about a potential donor and whether it made any difference to recipients. He found an overwhelmingly negative response to the idea of a murderer's heart. When I first read about it, I wondered if I would accept a murderer's heart? And afterwards, if my feelings about having a murderer's heart went on to change my personality, would the source of that change be relevant?

Medics are sceptical about most things, including the idea that the heart houses memory, and the evidence supports this: the heart is simply a bunch of nerves, muscles and chemicals. A study of forty-seven heart-transplant patients like Aaron found that although 15 per cent of patients felt their personality had changed following transplantation, even that was attributable to having suffered and survived a life-threatening event, and most other information related to the heart housing – or being linked to – emotion is completely anecdotal.

But art, literature and philosophy have been searching for greater meaning about the heart for more than 4,000 years, since ancient Egyptians believed that the heart symbolised truth; after death, they would weigh the heart against a feather of truth, to be eaten by a demon if the scales did not balance, leaving the person's soul restless for eternity. In this post-truth world, I wonder what will happen to our souls. We have nothing to weigh our hearts against.

Nurses do not explicitly search for meaning, but meaning is part and parcel of their day job. Nurses certainly use the language of the heart. They understand and describe patients as broken-hearted. Many nurses have seen it. And the best nursing comes from the heart, and not from the head.

Aaron gets me to help him write a letter to the mother of the boy who died and gave him his heart. The letter must not go directly, but the organ-donation coordinator is going to find out if the mother wants to read such a letter and, if so, will facilitate the anonymous handover at an appropriate time. Twenty years have passed since I helped Aaron write that letter, but I still remember the lines he wrote, which made me laugh: 'Did your son like strawberry ice-cream?' And cry: 'It's not fair that your son died so I can live. I absolutely promise I will never forget him.'

I think of the look that I noticed passing between the scrub nurse and the organ-donation coordinator. I think about how nursing is sometimes scrubbing in, passing the surgeon instruments and counting the swabs. Sometimes nursing is doing up the ties on the surgeon's gown, while other days it is handing the surgeon the instrument she or he hasn't yet asked for. And at other times it is recognising sadness and loss, and helping a teenage boy write a difficult letter.

At the end of my shift Aaron's mum tells me that he has always liked strawberry ice-cream, but they have avoided dairy food as it increased his symptoms of mucus production.

His mum smiles a thousand smiles. 'Aaron can have as much strawberry ice-cream as he wants now.'

7

To Live is So Startling

Where there is love there is no darkness.

Burundian proverb

The Nursing & Midwifery Code of Professional Conduct has a list of rules that nurses must live by. And I take them very seriously. But of course a number of times I find myself either knowingly or unknowingly deviating from the rules, and confidentiality has always been the trickiest aspect of the code, for a massive over-sharer like me. But, as a nurse, I am driven by the rule book and find comfort in ensuring that I maintain professionalism and standards, as set out by the Nursing & Midwifery Council (NMC):

5.1 Respect a person's right to privacy in all aspects of their care.

Nurses and midwives owe a duty of confidentiality to all those who are receiving care. This includes making sure that they are informed about their care, and that information about them is shared appropriately.

I am always careful about sharing information concerning patients, but I find myself working in another hospital as a qualified nurse on placement, while studying for a specialist qualification. The patient I am looking after is post-liver surgery, and I learn very quickly that liver-disease patients bleed in a way you cannot imagine. It's harrowing and I'm outside my comfort zone, but the nurses are totally relaxed. 'Too relaxed,' I think to myself, as one of them flicks through an Argos catalogue, and another orders a takeaway during our night shift. I take a higher moral ground, stay with my patient all evening and refuse the snacks they pass around. What kind of place is this?

It is with horror that I notice blood patterning my patient's charts – all over them. I wipe it off, and call over the nurse in charge. 'Somebody has left blood here,' I say. 'Imagine if a relative had seen it!'

She looks down, then smiles. 'Oh, that's not blood. That's Viennetta. Our lead consultant was eating a Viennetta during ward round, and it fell out of his mouth.'

I stand for many seconds, simply unable to speak. Of course I don't know it then, but that Viennetta-eater goes on to become my partner, and the father of my children.

Later in the shift a more sensible-looking consultant arrives. Thank goodness! He has a pristine white coat. He appears earnest, wandering around and checking on all the patients. The nurses at the nurses' station are all knee-deep in the catalogue when he looks at me.

'Shall I take you around?' I ask.

He nods. 'That would be great.'

I walk between all the patients on the unit, describing their conditions and treatment plans, giving him the necessary information from their files. He looks at the charts and then at the patients, before moving on to the next. Finally we get to my patient. I am tempted to tell him about the awful consultant who felt it appropriate to eat a Viennetta during ward round, when the nurse in charge shouts over to me. She is scary. The doctor says thank you, and disappears off. I do not blame him.

She walks over with a frown cutting her head in two. 'What were you telling him?' she asks.

'Well, you were all busy. So I updated him. Did a mini-ward round.'

She groans. 'Oh God. I'll have to do an incident form.'

'What do you mean?'

'He's not a doctor.'

I look at the door that has closed behind him. 'He is a doctor. He had a white coat. And what else would he be doing here?'

She points at the nurses' station, where large polystyrene packets are being opened by the nurses: chicken legs and buckets of chicken wings. 'He's from the takeaway.'

My mouth drops open as if it, too, is full of too much Viennetta.

'He's the chicken man.'

*

I fall in love with the Viennetta-eater, but not with surgical nursing. Surgery, it turns out, is my least-favourite type of nursing, for a number of reasons. I don't like the inconsistency in the workload, and the sudden change of pace. From when I worked on the neurosurgical unit, to looking after babies following complex heart surgery, I never quite get used to the extremes of activity: the immediate post-operative period, when a surgical patient requires intensive care, then the days of simple, quiet recovery. It can even be boring. But things can change in surgical nursing so suddenly it's hard to draw breath. Patients bleed to death very quickly and, following any surgery, there can be bleeding internally, requiring an immediate trip back to theatre in order that the surgeon can fix the problem. Outcomes for surgical patients are almost entirely dependent on the skill of the surgeon, and although the nurses can make an important difference to the patient's experience, it is the surgery itself that will or won't work.

But there are always exceptions. My friend, Gabby, is a senior staff nurse on the surgical ward. Nursing grading systems are based on a pay scale known as 'bands'. They begin at band 5 for a newly qualified staff nurse, and rise to band 8, which is a consultant nurse or similar. Gabby is band 6, but will no doubt be rising up the scale to reach management level before long. Usually in charge of a shift, she is the kind of person who would make a good military strategist. She has an overview of every single thing on her ward and plans the days meticulously, replanning with every outcome and unexpected event.

Surgical nursing is about managing potential complications and unexpected events. Surgical nurses are risk managers, strategists and ship-shape prioritisers. A surgical nurse needs to be excellent at assessing – a constant watcher for any change. Most bleeding, for example, happens internally, with few outward signs at first. A surgical nurse will know to look for a shiny abdomen, and will be assertive enough to get the surgeon out of theatre to come and assess the patient. Experienced surgical nurses know that conversations and escalations, and the right language to alert the surgeon to a problem, can save lives.

Mr Webb is a sixty-eight-year-old man who is on the surgical ward for a hemicolectomy, whereby part of the colon is removed to treat bowel cancer. The ward is full of Mr Webbs. The nurses on this surgical ward, where Gabby works, all seem brilliant. There is a definite culture on wards of leadership, mentoring and coaching: find the nurse in charge and the ward sister, to understand how kind the nurses will be. The surgery is important. And so is the aftermath. There is a stoma-care nurse, who becomes so important for patients who have to have a colostomy bag following surgery. Her job is a practical one, demonstrating how to care for a stoma, change the bag, manage things, and much, much more than that. She provides counselling and psychological support for what must be such a difficult experience. Mr Webb, however, doesn't need a stoma-care nurse. His cancer was taken out without the need for a colostomy bag, and the surgery went very well. But the day after the surgery his wife shouts out for help. 'He's not right,' she says.

Gabby hears the particular tone of her voice, knows the family well enough to take it seriously, drops everything she's doing and goes straight over to Mr Webb. She glances at his abdomen (not shiny), drains (not full) and colour (not great). Before she has even assessed him, she has asked the bedside nurse to get the doctor from the office. Mr Webb's breathing is odd. He is breathing in a funny rhythm, fast and then slow. And he is making strange cycling movements with his legs. As she tries to talk to him, Gabby notices his face is not symmetrical. Mr Webb is only making sounds, unable to respond properly.

By the time the doctor arrives minutes later, Gabby has spoken to Mrs Webb. 'I know this all seems incredibly frightening and there will be lots of activity around the bed, but it's very important that we assess your husband and get treatment for him quickly, if he needs it.'

Mrs Webb asks repeatedly about her husband's face.

'It is too soon to say,' says Gabby. She puts her arm around Mrs Webb briefly, before increasing Mr Webb's oxygen levels. 'Can you put a crash call out,' she tells another nurse.

By the time the resuscitation team arrives, Mr Webb is showing even more worrying posturing and erratic breathing. His wife is on the phone, crying, standing at the end of his bed. I hear her voice between sobs. 'But he was fine, they said he was fine.'

A doctor inserts a nasopharyngeal tube into Mr Webb's nose to keep his airways open. Mr Webb does not try, or doesn't have the physical capacity, to pull it out: a worrying sign. Gabby takes Mrs Webb to the office to explain things, and to keep her from having to witness all the needles and sudden management and scans her husband needs. Mr Webb's scan reveals a stroke. Treatment choices are difficult: some of the drugs used to treat strokes can cause bleeding, and Mr Webb is further at risk because of his recent surgery. However, he is still taken to a hyper-acute stroke unit for possible treatment or conservative management, where the experts will make a decision.

He is lucky. Hyper-acute stroke units are shown to reduce death rates and long-term disability. Around half of people who have a stroke live for less than one year. According to a recent Stroke Association report, there are 100,000 strokes in the UK every year, equating to someone having a stroke every five minutes.

Medical patients improve slowly, or else have a steady decline, and the nursing on medical wards is completely different from that on surgical wards. The landscape of the ward is the same: a long room with a nurses' station in the middle, patient and staff toilets on either side, a bathroom with a red emergency-call bell, a crash trolley next to a large notes trolley, an equipment room containing commodes and hoists and drip-stands, a dirty utility room, a treatment room, a relatives' room. But whereas the general surgical ward is on the fourth floor, next to theatres and recovery and intensive care, the medical ward is on the tenth floor. The lift takes ages to arrive. It stops at almost every level: a pregnant woman getting out on fifth for maternity; a family filing out on floor six for neurology. A doctor carrying a clipboard leaves at floor seven: the cardiac wards. A woman exits on level eight for the respiratory units, and another on level nine for the ear, nose and throat ward. A man with a jelly-like patch over his eye is clearly heading for the ophthalmology clinic above.

Medical wards are the nuts and bolts of a hospital. Surgery is where a complication like a stroke might happen, whereas the medical ward is where the long-term recovery must take place. Medical nursing can be acute or chronic, but is all in the details. And just as a physician is different from a surgeon, so a medical nurse is different from a surgical nurse, from a healthcare assistant, from a resuscitation nurse. Of course the principles are the same, but nursing is a language with different accents.

I am enjoying my work as a resuscitation nurse, which allows me to see all manner of patients and to travel around the hospital. I work short days now; normal days for most people, but short for nurses. It is not a traditional nursing role, though increasingly the traditional aspects of nursing are being given over to unqualified nurses. Nurses' and junior doctors' lines are blurring, and advanced nursing roles are being driven by a political agenda that concerns not necessarily what is right for the patient, but financial savings. It is cheaper to have a nurse perform the tasks that a registrar might previously have performed. Nurses put in drips, take bloods, analyse blood results, even intubate and insert arterial lines; they have their own anaesthetic lists and, in some areas, are on the doctors' rota, with nurse-led retrievals of sick patients.

There are nurse-led clinics, and nurse practitioners caring for adult patients needing transfers on ECMO. Nurses are diagnosing, treating, prescribing, leading cardiac-arrest teams, and teaching and assessing consultants on advanced life-support courses. And they are paid as nurses. But the real expense comes in the tasks at the heart of nursing: changing beds, taking observations, helping a person drink their tea or use the toilet, or listening to their stories. There is a danger of forgetting what nursing is, what it means: the importance of providing care. The jobs that a nurse would traditionally do are often passed on to healthcare assistants. Certainly on this ward, aside from visitors like me, the infection-control nurse, a pharmacist and the hairdresser, all I can see are healthcare assistants: un-qualified nurses working for as little as £7.87 an hour. The minimum wage is £7.50 an hour. The hospital advises that the role of nursing or healthcare assistant includes: washing and dressing patients, helping to feed patients, toileting, making them more comfortable. These tasks lie at the heart of nursing on most wards and are often the most important aspects of the patient's care and experience. Kindness, empathy, compassion and providing dignity. This is what makes a good nurse.

Gladys is in a bed on the medical ward and shouts every few minutes. She refused the commode earlier and now she screams, 'I've shit, I've shit' to the healthcare assistants, who rush over, rolling up their sleeves.

'Any chance you can give us a hand?' Fatima asks me, pulling the curtain round.

Changing a bed: what a thing to do for someone. The smell makes my eyes water. You get used to all sorts of smells, as a nurse. But having spent most of my time as a children's nurse, I've never got used to the violence with which adults vomit and shit and bleed. I have to leave the room on one occasion and feel terrible about it for evermore, when, due to an abdominal blockage, a man vomits his own faeces. Sick people have colostomy bags that need changing; and ileostomies (a stoma in the small intestine); and spew thick green secretions from their tracheostomies; have yellow penile or grey vaginal discharge; pass melaena from their rectums, the foulest-smelling thing of all, from a bleed in a stomach. They have infected gastrostomies and ulcerated legs; pressure sores big enough to fit a fist in, with the bone visible. They ooze green pus – and have cyst-filled lesions that burst open – a year-old mayonnaise-smelling glue. Or, as in my case, when I had a bowling-ball-sized growth filled with hair and teeth and bones removed with an ovary, they have disgusting variations of standard gestational cell growth. And it is the nurse, or nursing assistant, who cleans, washes, dresses, disposes of body fluid, opens the windows and sprays air freshener.

But for all that I've seen and touched and smelled, and as difficult as it is at the time, there is a patient at the centre of it, afraid and embarrassed. Nurses make good poker players, understanding the importance of not breathing in; of breath-holding so subtly that the patient does not realise, and does not see any expression other than a matter-of-fact one. The horror of our bodies – our humanity, our flesh and blood – is something nurses must bear, lest the patient think too deeply, remember the lack of dignity that makes us all vulnerable. It is our vulnerability that unites us. Promoting dignity in the face of illness is one of the best gifts a nurse can give. I am reminded of the very beginning of the Nursing & Midwifery Code of Professional Conduct, clause 1.1: nurses must 'treat patients with kindness, respect and compassion'.

Dignity has been much written about, from a philosophical perspective. Immanuel Kant, for example, described the inherent and equal worth of every individual. And dignity is central to most religious beliefs, with the Protestant and Catholic Churches both citing that all human beings, created in the image of God, have dignity. In Islam the Prophet Muhammad is also reported to have said that Adam was created in God's image. And human dignity, or *kevod ha-beriyot*, is also a central consideration of Judaism. Dignity and nobility are part of each human's birth-right. Dignity is political, too. The United Nations Universal Declaration of Human Rights states that 'All human beings are born free and equal in dignity and rights.' Loss of respect for fellow human beings, and the removal of dignity, has in the past led to the dehumanisation at the heart of genocide.

'I've shit, I've shit.' Gladys keeps talking. She is clearly distressed, her body arching and twisting, and further spreading the mess and smell. She is covered in faeces. I remember my early nursing days when I studied the Bristol stool-scale, a pictorial poster showing different kinds of stool and assessing the severity of abnormality. But charts and guidelines and scales don't prepare you for real life. Gladys has every type of stool described on the Bristol scale, all at once. There are lumps, blobs, ragged edges and the liquid has spilled over the incontinence pad, up her back and onto the pillow. There are flecks of green in her hair. Globs of it spray around the place, threatening to land on our faces, too. It is all I can manage not to retch.

'Gladys, we are here to help you.' Fatima has filled a bowl with warm soapy water and dips her elbow into it, as if testing a baby's bath. Gladys watches and becomes still, as if this triggers a memory somewhere. Like many people, Gladys has dementia. It is estimated that by 2021 the number of people with dementia in the UK will have reached one million. Dementia is a cruel disease, causing memory loss and changes in personality, confusion and hallucinations. It must be like living in a terrible nightmare.

Gladys keeps asking for her friend, Doffy, her memory caught elsewhere, dipping in and out of her life, with no clear order. Fatima later tells me that Doffy lives in Australia and that she and Gladys used to work together as cooks in a school kitchen sixty years ago. The more distressed Gladys becomes, the further back she goes. You can never physically go home, because every time you leave, there are new experiences that change you. But with dementia you can sort of go home, be totally present in a former time in life. A strange comfort during a terrifying experience.

'Doffy, is she here yet? We'll be late. What time is it?'

I place one of Gladys's legs over the other, and my hands on her hip and shoulder, and roll her gently towards me. Nurses all develop back pain. Back injury and pain account for 40 per cent of all sickness in the NHS, at a cost of £400 million for nurses' sick days alone; almost £1 billion, if you include healthcare assistants. Musculoskeletal injuries occur when you lift or move patients. And nursing is heavy work. Of course trusts now have extensive training and equipment for nurses, in order that manual handling of patients is kept to a minimum and the hospital is not sued if something goes wrong. But when the staffing is as bad as it is here today, there is nobody to help move a patient who has been incontinent or find another hoist, as the hoist has broken and there isn't time to report it. And when a person's muscles don't work, due to illness, medication or wastage, the nurse must act as the muscles for them, risking her own musculoskeletal system in small actions that are repeated often: holding Gladys a fraction too long while Fatima fills the water. When Gladys jerks suddenly, I don't let her fall, as we are taught. Her face is full of shame and distress and, although my back twinges, I judge in a second that the harm I would do this poor woman by letting her fall back into all the faeces is worth my pain. One day I might be Gladys. You might.

Gladys's skin is delicate and I need to be careful that it doesn't break. The smallest of unhealed cuts can become pressure sores, bruises and wounds. Her face, hovering at my abdomen, looks up at me, as Fatima begins washing her. She has a large yellow clinical waste bag and a pack of soft wipes. She uses nearly half a pack, the bin filling up with soiled wipes, the water in the bowl becoming dirtier.

'You okay there, Gladys?' she asks. 'Won't be long and we'll have you comfortable.' She disappears to empty the bowl in the toilet, and returns with it refilled with clean and soapy water. She dips her elbow in once more, before a second wash of Gladys's back and straightening the sheet taut, lest a small ridge or rumpled section causes skin problems. We roll Gladys back and rearrange her pillows, then raise the bed slightly.

I glance at my watch, stay a while. Gladys still has tight hold of my hand. She looks out of the window. Far away. She has stopped shouting and her breathing is regular and calm. She smells of a newborn baby.

For a few moments Gladys seems coherent. She says thank you. 'I feel much better. We're not late. Ready in time and Doffy will be here any minute. Can't let those kids go hungry.' She glances back out past the other beds, the smudged dirty window, to the sky. 'What time is it? Is she coming soon?'

I tell her it's almost five.

'Really? That late in the day already? How time flies.' She looks at me. 'How time flies.'

I have looked after patients on the surgical wards, the medical wards and the mental-health unit, babies and children and women giving birth. But it turns out that my favourite kind of nursing is a complex mixture of all specialities: surgical, medical, paediatric, adult, and mental health. It is in intensive care that I find my home. There I meet Tommy.

Tommy does not want to see the sun. 'It's a lovely view,' I say, looking out of the window. We are up on the ninth floor in one of the side-rooms in the middle of the ward and the sunrise over smoggy London is incredible. But Tommy closes his eyes whenever I open the curtains, and screws his face up tightly. Tommy is nine years old and paralysed from the neck down, following a road-traffic accident in which he broke his neck and his pelvis. He has a tracheostomy, so the words and sounds from his mouth cannot be heard, but instead a rasping intake of air over and over again and the sight of Tommy's sobbing face.

I look after Tommy for many consecutive nights over many months. Twelve-and-a-half hours when it's often simply me and him. Tommy has spiky black hair, which his dad puts gel in every morning, until Tommy's pillow is patterned with sticky blotches. Next to his bed is a small table with a photograph of Tommy, his mum, dad and cousins on holiday, drinking through long curly straws from coconuts. Another photo of a cat wearing a studded collar. A small radio set to Kiss FM. A pile of books, each stamped on the inside 'Greystone Junior School Library', and each past the due-back date. His mum watches me leafing through them. 'It's a great school,' she says. 'And Tommy is supersmart. Straight-A student. Not like me. I failed my O levels. But he's heading for Oxford, aren't you, Tom? And football mad, like his dad.' I watch her swallow. Look at her husband, then Tommy.

Tommy blinks slowly, then starts to cry.

I wonder what he was like before. I always try and imagine the lives of the patients I care for, search for clues that help me nurse them. I try and imagine what the situation will do to the entire picture. Tommy's dad's job, which takes him away to oil rigs for weeks at a time. His mother's support network. Their relationship, resilience and expectations.

Nursing Tommy means I will need all the clues I can get in order to help him and his family. It is a series of steady tasks. Every hour, on the hour, I document his observations and his ventilator settings and write them all on a large poster-sized chart in different-coloured pens. I join the dots, look for patterns: the temperature line going up, the blood pressure climbing. Spinal-cord patients like Tommy are at risk of autonomic dysreflexia, which is an abnormal physiological response to damaged spinal nerves, resulting in severe hypertension. It can be caused by something as straightforward as constipation or a kink in a urinary catheter, and so good nursing care is essential. I watch him closely to prevent and recognise this life-threatening emergency. Nursing Tommy involves intimate care, too. I wash him, roll him, ensure he is not staying in one position for too long, as he is at risk of developing pressure sores. Tommy's body is now stabilised, though he is full of metalwork holding him together, and he will need more surgery on his pelvis in the future. Everything is fragile. Details make all the difference. I make sure his socks are not scrunched up, for example, on a regular basis. A simple thing, but it could have devastating consequences, particularly as his resistance to infections such as MRSA is so poor. I deliver his food: Tommy cannot currently eat orally, so I hang up giant bags of milk-like feed that go directly into a tube inside his stomach called a gastrostomy. I administer medication through this tube, too.

But although I provide all this physical care for Tommy, it is his mind that needs nursing most of all. It is mental-health nursing that I perform for him, despite the appearance of physical tasks. The most helpful task of all is to build a trusting and therapeutic relationship with Tommy and listen to him. Really listen.

We talk through feelings. 'I am not surprised,' I tell him, when he mouths that he wants to go home. 'I think I would feel the same. You must really miss the time before the accident.'

He is closed-mouthed for a while. Nobody has said this to him yet. They have told him it will be soon, that he will be able to go home and see his bedroom and his friends when he is well enough. But I listen properly. I understand his desire to go home is a desire to travel back in time to his old life. He is not talking about a physical home.

'But I hope you won't always feel like this. In fact, I am sure of it. It's a terrible thing to happen. I can't even imagine how you must feel. And I'll do anything I can to make it even a fraction better. Take each hour with you. Each second.' I stroke his hair as I speak. 'I am with you. Right here, all through the night.' It is not enough, but it's all I have.

I read to Tommy that night, and many others when he can't sleep, his eyes open too wide in the near-darkness. We read *Harry Potter* and, as the story develops, his eyes close a little: he escapes a fraction. He requires ventilating – his broken neck means he can no longer breathe unaided – and so he is on the intensive-care ward, even though he is by now stable; Tommy has such complex needs that it may take many months before he gets out – years even before he gets to his physical home. He develops pseudomonas and his neck smells of a sewer. There is green pus coming from his tracheostomy wound; he coughs green phlegm; has a colostomy bag and a urinary catheter.

I sit outside his room and listen to the chug of machinery, Tommy's metamorphosis into a hybrid human, reliant on technology, able to move only his head. The whole world feels cruel. I listen to his mum and wonder how on earth she will cope. She is a single parent much of the time when Tommy's dad is working away. Tommy's mum also suffers with depression. 'She's been wobbly for ages,' his dad tells me. 'We've been in a bad place. But maybe something like this puts everything into perspective. This kind of thing brings people closer. You don't realise how lucky you are until something like this happens.' I try to let my head agree with him but it knows better. Tommy's accident can't fix his mum. A severely sick child will only be more pressure on her fragile mental health. On their finances. On their relationship. A sick child is the first domino to fall.

Tommy's tenth birthday arrives while he is on the ward. The nurses decorate his bed space with tinsel leftover from Christmas and found in the bottom cupboard of the staff kitchen. They stick cards along his metal bed edges and ventilator with surgical tape, and one nurse brings in some balloons that she had bought and filled with helium on her day off. But the balloons look sad under the stark lights of the intensive-care ward; too bright, too plastic, everything – even life – seems artificial. Tracy, one of the most experienced PICU nurses, brings in some flowers from her garden, a mishmash of colours and sizes, straggly and rugged, and puts them in a small plastic cup on top of the ventilator. 'That's better,' I say. 'Look at those gorgeous flowers, Tommy. How beautiful.' Tommy looks at them but then closes his eyes.

The nurse in charge today walks past. 'You can't have flowers there, Trace, totally banned.'

Tracy humphs and moves the flowers from the top of the ventilator to the desk nearby. I watch her lean over to Tommy. 'My boy deserves flowers on his birthday,' she says, kissing her fingers then touching his cheek. 'Double figures. Ten years old and a heartbreaker already.' She loves him. We all do. He's been with us for so long by now. But Tracy loves him the most. She talks to him all day, as she washes him, rubs cream into his skin, stretches his legs out, the radio in the background with football matches or dance music. She dances, terribly, punching her hands in the air. It is the only time I see Tommy laugh.

There is a mound of presents at the bottom of Tommy's bed. Many are from the nurses but his dad has a large sack of gifts when he walks in. 'There's the birthday boy!' He kisses Tommy's face and they smile at one another. 'You've done well this year.' He starts pulling out presents one by one and piling them on the bed until Tommy is wide-eyed.

When Tommy falls asleep his parents stay on the ward. 'He wanted a bike,' his mum says. 'I always promised him that he'd get one on his tenth birthday. For years he's been asking for a bike. I didn't want to spoil him. Told him he'd need to wait, that it was a special present so it had to come on an extra special birthday. And only if he was good.' Her body folds in half. She holds her stomach.

I touch her shoulders. 'I'm so sorry,' I say. The tears I am holding in burn my eyes. The pain she feels should not be experienced by any human being.

Tommy's dad puts his arm around her and squeezes. 'It's temporary. That's what I think anyway. He's a fighter,' he says. 'I know he'll walk again. I just know it, love. Doctors get things wrong all the time. And you hear about all sorts of treatments in America. I'll work double shifts if I have to, to pay for it. He'll be back on the football pitch in no time, won't he?'

He looks over at Tommy, who's asleep surrounded by equipment and machinery. Tommy's mum stares straight through me. But his dad turns to me and nods the kind of slow nod you do when you want someone to agree with you.

But all I can do is push my razorblade tears even further back in my head. Fake a smile. I look away, and focus on Tracy's wild flowers. The colours of nature.

8

Small Things, with Great Love

Life is occupied in both perpetuating itself and in surpassing itself; if all it does is maintain itself, then living is only not dying.

Simone de Beauvoir

I watch the mother's face mostly, details I hadn't noticed before: the slope of her eyebrows, the clenching of her teeth, eyes rimmed with red. But it is Rhianna's granddad who looks to be carrying the most grief. His face is unironed linen, folded in and crumpled over.

Rhianna is a talented singer, dancer and actor. She has been attending a local theatre-arts school since she was two, and spends her spare time watching musicals with her granddad, who lives nearby. She regularly visits him after school and they rush through her homework in order to sit down to early Elvis films, or *South Pacific, My Fair Lady, Mary Poppins*. Her mum tells me that Rhianna's bedroom at home is full of memorabilia that he's given her, from his days 'tapping the boards': ticket stubs from shows he's seen, old dance-shoes tied together with their frayed laces, hanging from hooks on her wall; a top hat that he wore in panto one season in Bognor Regis; a framed certificate in stage lighting; the original umbrella – he tells her it was one of many – from *Singin' in the Rain*.

Rhianna has a large wardrobe full of costumes from shows gone by, attended every single time by her granddad: glittery leotards that leave a layer of gold flecks on her carpet, a jade-green mermaid dress, a white layered tutu. Her quilt has tiny ballerinas dancing across it, and next to her bed is her most prized possession: a tiny wind-up musical box, a dancing figure spinning on top, which Rhianna liked to wind up every morning as she woke: a ritual that became background noise to her parents.

It is the lack of the music box being wound up that first alerts her mum that something is wrong. The mornings are silent. There is none of the tinny tinkling that usually greets them, coming from Rhianna's room. When they go in, they notice that she is still fast asleep, sleeping longer and yet more tired. They put it down to the number of times Rhianna seems to wake in the night to use the toilet. 'Stop drinking so much milk before bed,' her mum tells her. But she is worried. Rhianna was always a tiny thing, but now her clothes are hanging off her.

One morning Rhianna begins to complain of tummy ache, feeling sick. Her granddad stays with her while her parents go to work. By the time her parents return, Rhianna is confused and doesn't appear to recognise them. Everything goes through her mum's mind. Rhianna is seven. Her room smells of nail-varnish remover. Did she take it from the bathroom and spill it? She may have inhaled fumes from painting her nails repeatedly. Or perhaps she's being bullied at school? Recently she even seemed to have lost interest in her love of singing, acting and dancing. For such a bubbly, confident girl, she had become very quiet. They fear they will never wake to the sound of the music box again.

I think of my own daughter's music box: the miniature ballerina that she delights in watching, her eyes wide, mesmerised.

Rhianna deteriorates even more, and by now her breathing is different, shallow, fast. The doctors in A&E work quickly, taking a history and blood tests. 'She has diabetes,' they tell her parents. Something called 'diabetic ketoacidosis' (DKA). They transfer her to the Paediatric Intensive-Care Unit, where Trisha and I meet Rhianna for the first time. Trisha is on a nurse orientation programme and arrived some months before from the Philippines. I am her mentor.

The transition between being a junior nurse and coached by senior staff, and becoming a mentor nurse and more experienced, is something I have barely noticed. It has crept up on me, though moving up nursing grades means taking responsibility for students and orientation programmes, and for nurses from other countries who have arrived in London following NHS recruitment drives in India, Europe or the Philippines. Mentoring a nurse from abroad is a different experience from mentoring a home-grown nurse. Most of the junior nurses from the Philippines that I've ever worked with were senior nurse-managers at home and have far more experience than I do. They smile anyway, when I tell them what they already know. We all understand that both nurses and doctors will learn good teamwork, not in a classroom, but by experiencing it; as Kant put it so well: 'There can be no doubt that all our knowledge begins with experience.'

'Diabetes is getting so common at home,' Trisha tells me.

'It's getting more common everywhere,' I say. 'Type-two anyway.' Diabetes was first discovered in the 1550s BC, when ancient healers noticed that ants were attracted to the urine of patients who were emaciated and urinating frequently. It is estimated that 3.9 million people in the UK alone are sufferers, and this number is going up at an alarming rate. There are some interesting developments in the treatment of type-2 diabetes, involving the venom from a giant lizard. A drug – exenatide – was approved for development in 2005. It is synthetic, although it is extracted from the Gila monster's saliva. Rhianna, though, is suffering from the rarer, and far more acutely dangerous, type-1 diabetes.

Rhianna's parents are distraught. 'We missed it. How could we have missed it? She was drinking so much milk. So thirsty. Eating loads. And losing weight.'

'It is not your fault,' I tell them repeatedly. 'You didn't cause this.' Rhianna is the only patient under my care. Usually in PICU there is one nurse to one patient. Rhianna needs various treatments: insulin infusion, fluid resuscitation, potassium, and careful monitoring, as the timings of the treatments themselves can cause fatal harm.

Her granddad doesn't speak, but his eyes are full of pain and guilt. He shakes his head every so often and watches Rhianna's quick breathing.

'We are monitoring her very closely, her observations and bloods. Checking her blood levels. The way she is breathing is because she's trying to blow off carbon dioxide, which is a good sign that she is fighting it.'

By the time a child with DKA decompensates, stops propping up physiology by keeping things like their blood pressure normal, they stop fighting and their chance of survival diminishes. Rhianna is compensating. Although it is terrifying for her granddad to watch, I am relieved to see her fast breathing. Her pH is the lowest I've ever seen. Acid-base balance is incredible; we are too acid or too alkaline close to death, and our body compensates to rectify it – our will to live. If the acid level is too great, we produce hydrogen ions to neutralise it, like sponges mopping up and absorbing a spillage. We can tell how sick a patient is, in the first instance, by how many sponges they have produced; how they perform, or not, on a cellular level – homeostasis. Human beings are so incredibly fragile, and we need our pH to stay within minuscule parameters: for example, our acid pH should be between 7.35 and 7.46. If a patient's pH is 6.8, it is incompatible with human life. Eventually we stop making sponges – we decompensate. We only have so much fight in us.

By all accounts, Rhianna's pH is incompatible with life; should it drop by a decimal point, then Rhianna will surely die. Her breathing is maintaining that decimal better than anything we can do using technology. A life-support machine would probably kill her. It is similarly dangerous when treating patients who suffer from asthma. Dusan, the senior consultant, teaches some junior doctors in a mini-teaching session, and I listen in: 'The minute we intubate, there is a risk of bilateral pneumothorasis, subcutaneous emphysema, hyper-inflation requiring a senior anaesthetist and early intervention.' I look at Tracy, who is standing next to me. 'What does all that mean?' I whisper.

She shrugs. 'We can put air in, but can't take it out.'

As with asthma, treating a child with DKA requires medicine and expert knowledge, of course, but also faith in nature. We are getting used to seeing the patient first, holistically, before simply correcting the numbers. Medical treatment for DKA used to involve wading in to correct the numbers, giving fluid and insulin and bicarbonate, before we realised that this aggressive treatment was making children's brains swell, hastening – if not causing – coma and death. DKA is now treated softly, slowly. We remember the dock leaf next to the stinging nettle. We let Rhianna breathe quickly, let her numbers look horrific, support nature as she stabilises. I stand guard against anyone who wants to intervene too much.

Trisha and I are working today in the bed space next to Tracy. Coming up to retirement age, Tracy has never wanted to move up the managerial or education nursing routes, instead choosing a lifetime of patient care, happy to stay at her pay grade. She has twenty years' more intensive-care experience than our most senior consultant, Dusan, who is standing at the nurses' station eating a croissant while looking at an X-ray.

A new doctor is writing up a prescription. He wanders over to Tracy's patient's ventilator and begins fiddling with the pressures. He adjusts the controls for tidal volume, the ventilator alarms and the patient's chest rises higher than before. Tracy moves quickly. First she slaps the doctor's hand away; next she turns the dials back to exactly where she had the settings, then checks the patient's breathing.

The newbie looks bewildered. 'This patient's CO_2 is rising,' he says.

'I'm well aware of that.' Tracy blocks the doctor from the ventilator controls with her body. She folds her arms. 'I'm planning to extubate him later.'

'We haven't discussed that on ward round.' The doctor looks confused. 'There's nothing planned, in his medical notes.'

Tracy laughs. She says nothing, but waves the doctor away with her hands.

He tries a different approach. 'I'll have to raise it with the consultant.'

'You do that,' she says. 'He's over there.'

In the UK it's the doctors – but usually the nurses really – who manage the weaning-off of a child from a life-support machine. In America and Canada, registered respiratory therapists are the ones who are trained to do this. Tracy doesn't have any specific qualifications to alter the ventilation. But, as with most nursing, I always judge skill based on who I would want to look after my family members. Tracy would be at the top.

The doctor humphs off and I watch him lean in to talk to Dusan, who pops the last of the croissant in his mouth. He puts his arm on the new doctor's shoulder, shakes his head, looks over at Tracy, smiles. They are old friends and have shared more than most of us see in a lifetime. They trust each other.

Tracy shakes her head. 'If the Hippocratic Oath is to "Do no harm", then a nurses' oath should be to make sure the doctors can fulfil their Hippocratic Oath.' She laughs. 'I think all junior doctors should spend a month as a nurse. We'd never have to clean a coffee cup left in the sink again, that's for sure.'

Rhianna's breathing becomes slower and deeper. She is developing Kussmaul breathing. Adolph Kussmaul was a nineteenth-century doctor who identified deep, laboured gasping as a sign of coma and imminent death. It looks terrifying – what people describe as 'air hunger'. Rhianna is barely conscious, biting the air in front of her. I think of the woman

I first saw giving birth. How we are born, how we die. Those times when we are most human are when we appear least so. Rhianna has her eyes rolled back, biting the air, her body contracting with each strange breath.

'Can she hear us?'

'I'm sure she can,' I lie.

But her mum can't think of what to say.

Her granddad begins talking. 'You need to get well soon,' he says. 'There is the end-of-year show coming up.'

'Will she be better?' her mum asks. 'How long will she be in intensive care?'

Diabetic ketoacidosis can lead to cerebral oedema (swelling of the brain), coma and death. If cerebral oedema occurs in children, as it has in Rhianna, approximately 58 per cent of children recover completely, 21 per cent survive with a degree of brain damage, and 21 per cent die.

Rhianna's mum keeps asking me questions about her recovery. Rhianna may not recover, but these are figures I keep to myself. I do not want to be dishonest, but I can see no benefit in telling her at this stage. I hope she will never need to know this. There is not much nursing I can do for Rhianna now. Only time will help, or not. But nursing means thinking ahead, even if the path in front is unthinkable. I move the furniture to the side of the room, check that the crash trolley is nearby; when her parents say they might pop out for a coffee, I suggest that Trisha makes them one instead, in case the doctors are coming to give an update. The room feels heavy, the air thick. The best nursing I can do is make sure the parents are with Rhianna if she dies, ensure they have spiritual support, that if the worst happens they get to say goodbye. The death of a child is unthinkable, but even more so a child dying alone.

'Is there anyone I can call, who you'd like to be with you all at this time?' I ask. 'Any family – or people from your community; your church, if you have one?'

Rhianna's brother visits. He's eight, all wide-eyed and slow-moving. He keeps his hands in his pockets, I notice. Trisha notices, too. It turns out that she has a son the same age, whom she has left in the Philippines with her mother so that she can come and earn money to send home, working as a nurse in the NHS. It is not uncommon: all of the Filipino nurses I've ever worked with have left children behind, to come and work in the NHS.

Trisha squats down at his level. 'Don't worry about touching anything. If you wash your hands, you could touch her hand, while I tell you what all the tubes are for.'

She takes him to the sink and helps him. When they return he is less wide-eyed.

Trisha laughs. 'She certainly does look strange, I'm sure. But she is getting better now, thanks to the fantastic doctors. Maybe you could be a doctor when you grow up.'

'I want to be a footballer.'

'Of course,' she says. She looks for a few seconds at the floor. 'Like my son.'

Rhianna is not on the High-Dependency Unit when I return for a day shift after a few days off. Her empty bed space is being cleaned for another patient. There are a few terrifying moments when you come back on shift and look for patients who were previously very sick, and you do not yet know whether or not the patient survived. Nurses never know, when they go home, if they will see the patient they have cared for the next morning. It is not something you can think about too much or the job would be impossible.

'Gone to the ward,' Dusan says. He is looking at an ECG on a monitor.

I'm glad Rhianna's family never needed the awful statistics that I held in my head. I never see Rhianna again, or her granddad or parents, but I often think of her, waking up next to an old music box, and imagine how the sound of that music must feel to her family when they hear it. I like to imagine her at her granddad's house, rushing through her homework in order to watch old films and dreaming of pop stardom. I am relieved that medical understanding of DKA has led to treatment that respects human physiology and compensatory mechanisms, and to caring for the whole person instead of simply trying to correct a set of numbers. Rhianna's brain recovered without injury; she is now truly living.

*

The other patients who remain in paediatric intensive care are either dying or not dying, but none are truly living. It is where people can't be looked after in slices. Where nursing means caring for the mental-health disorder exhibited by a parent, exacerbated by their child's serious illness, while looking post-operatively after a child who has an underlying medical disease and a learning disability. It is everything, and every single day is completely different.

The PICU where I am working is on the ninth floor of the hospital, in Panda Wing. It looks futuristic, one parent remarks: 'It's like the *Starship Enterprise*.' This is a place of strange quiet, a level hum of the machines and a rhythmic lulling of the ventilators. Luckily, intensive care is an area of the hospital that most of us can avoid. The children receive life support, often for multi-organ failure, while they recover from critical illness. The unit is totally different from A&E. Everything here is controlled and organised (intensive-care nurses – like me – are often control freaks), and there are advanced machines surrounding each bed space: ventilators to take over the patient's breathing, sometimes even ECMO (a machine that acts as a patient's heart and lungs and circulates the blood outside the patient's body, oxygenating it and returning it the reddest of red, the last streak of sunset).

The child lies at the centre of it all, oblivious, sedated and sometimes pharmacologically paralysed. Awash with tubes doing different jobs: ET tube in the mouth or nose; NG tube leading to the stomach; CVP line in the jugular vein, fanning out of the patient's neck like grotesque peacock feathers; arterial line measuring blood pressure, and allowing regular blood samples to check the fractional numbers that tell the team everything. An experienced intensive-care nurse can predict the numbers before the blood enters the blood-gas-analysis machine. She will tell the doctor the level of oxygen simply by the shade of red.

There are light-boxes above the desks to show X-rays and centralised computer screens, enabling the nurses to monitor all the vital signs of the patients in PICU in detail. Nobody ever does this. There is never time to sit down at the nurses' station. They sit – if they have to input obser-vations on the computers or make notes – right next to their patients. An invisible thread keeps them there, near to the endless things that can go wrong. But most of the time they are standing, checking the many machines that keep their patient alive, tidying the bed space, keeping the computerised notes, the prescription charts, the prescrip-tions themselves; emptying drains, changing syringes of inotropes, checking ventilator settings; talking to the families.

There is sometimes a runner: each patient needs their own nurse for round-the-clock care, and the runner might fetch equipment or medication, or help with cares, turns, bed changes, dressing changes, checking infusions, double-checking blood transfusions or controlled drugs. But increasingly, as PICU is stretched and squeezed, there is no such person available. When the bedside nurses need to use the toilet or take a break, the nurse in the next bed has to care for two patients at once, and the likelihood of mistakes or emergencies increases. Nurses time the sedation carefully. And the nurse in charge is expert at decision-making about skill mix: which nurse is placed next to which patient; which child is likely to require greater skill and experience, become sicker or more unstable. Nurses become expert at predicting who will deteriorate, based not on their numbers, but on the instincts of the nurse in charge. A strange kind of telepathy.

It's always busy, but today there is no time to get the ward straight and there are piles of items everywhere, half-cleaned, but not properly: gauze squares on the floor, empty cardboard trays piled up next to the bin, boxes of gloves bursting open, reaching out. There is a blocked toilet with a sign on it, and a maintenance job number written on the whiteboard. Maintenance staff in the hospital also triage jobs. Urgent jobs that might involve risk are prioritised: smoke coming through an air vent brought them running, before the fire department. A fire in PICU would be a total disaster. Hospitals plan for it as best they can, and nurses have annual fire training where the question of PICU comes up:

'What if you can't move a patient?'

'Leave them.'

'What if you have more patients than you have portable ventilators and oxygen?'

'Take those less sick first.'

'What about the others?'

A line of ventilators in the treatment room waits to be set up with tubing and checked by the technician or nurse. The haemofiltration machines pull off waste products from a patient's blood, then replacement fluid is added and the blood is returned to the patient, doing the job of a patient's kidneys. Giovanni Alfonso Borelli (1608–79) was a Neapolitan mathematician whose famous work *De Motu Animalium* ('On the Movement of Animals') recognises the mechanism of filtration: 'Urine is separated from the blood in the kidneys mechanically as a result of the narrowness and configuration of the vessels.'

Understanding the kidneys, and nursing children requiring haemofiltration, to this day requires mathematics. Large bags of filtration fluid lie at the bottom of the machines on special scales, like the weighing-in area of a self-service supermarket checkout, to ensure the patient's circulating blood volume is balanced. The fluid-balance charts that the nurses fill in are extremely complicated and important. The bags of waste products are a colour somewhere between straw and out-of-date mustard. What goes out must go back in. Yet they are not foolproof. A nurse I worked with once accidentally put her handbag on these special scales, which caused the machine to rapidly begin taking off too much blood through the vascath. The vascath is a large catheter in the patient's internal jugular vein. 'Flush the vascath, quick – flush the vascath' is a sentence that no nurse in charge wants to hear shouted across the ward.

Working on paediatric intensive care gives a lifetime of perspective. A difficult day means that a child dies, and those caring for that child are left wondering if they could have done something differently, if they missed something – or, worse, if there was anything they did to contribute to the child's death. 'A difficult day on PICU is not when a child dies, but when you accidentally kill one,' a doctor half-jokes to me. We look after children who haunt us for ever, as we go over our actions, wearing our mistakes like a coat. Everyone knows that a dinner party with medical professionals will often result in gruesome conversations or a sick sense of humour, a result of coping mechanisms developed over the years. Daily life demands it. But despite our best efforts to cope, certain patients stay with us.

Some cases, I'm sure – although nurses never admit it or get treated for it – cause post-traumatic stress disorder in the carers. Nurses and doctors, like patients, do not always cope, but instead simply survive. Maintaining morale among nurses and doctors was identified by Goran Haglund, the Swedish anaesthetist who opened the first PICU in 1955, as one of the important difficulties of PICU. Freud thought of morale as being rooted in the horizontal ties between members of a group who had all put the same leader in command, replacing their ego ideal (the inner image of oneself as one wants to become). I have a discussion with Dusan about the God-complex of another consultant we know. 'If you're in charge of everything in a hierarchical system, then what happens to your own morale? If you are at the top of the food chain and every decision rests with you, what happens to your own ego?'

Morale seems to affect nurses and doctors differently, and the doctors I work with on PICU seem better able – or have developed mechanisms that are healthy or otherwise – to suppress emotional fallout. Some recent research highlights that nurses are particularly vulnerable to moral distress. In a strange way I am glad. It is when you no longer feel pain that you suffer the worst injuries.

But I am developing my own coping mechanisms. Most days I go home and forget about the children I've looked after. Like people in other jobs, I can usually leave work at work. But today is going to be a difficult day. Mahesh is seventeen years old, suffers from muscular dystrophy and needs a life-support machine to breathe. Mahesh and I become more than patient and nurse; we become friends. He is funny, and he has nicknames for all of us that – unable to speak – he writes down in shaky handwriting. Mine is Scruff (I always have a pen stuck in my ponytail, scuffed shoes, door codes and timings scribbled on the back of my hand). Mahesh is at the end of his life. I nurse him in a side-room. He and his family have made the agonising decision that he will not have a tracheostomy and he will not be re-intubated with a breathing tube in his mouth, or have a breathing tube put in his trachea any more. Mahesh's anatomy would not allow it anyway: his breathing tube is the smallest we have, barely allowing air in and out from the life-support machine. His family are in the process of saying goodbye, spending the last few weeks with him.

I have one job and that is to keep Mahesh comfortable, and make sure above all else that his precarious breathing tube does not come out. If it does, he will die, as the family have decided that another tube would not be put into his neck. I have to be careful. I watch his tube obsessively, not allowing anyone to move him or turn him without my holding onto it. Every morning I change the tapes to keep them clean and dry and secure his tube. The tube must not fall out. A simple nursing task: to change tapes on a tube and secure them. Like most nursing tasks; like kindness itself – simple and extremely important.

One day I cut the old tapes, ready with the new ones. But it isn't the tapes I have cut. It is the tube itself: the cuff that holds the tube in place. I have cut through the plastic.

It is that moment just after you have cut yourself and the blood appears. Before I know how bad things really are. The seconds in between. But it is only a few seconds before the alarms, the whooshing of air leaking, the look on Mahesh's twisting face as he struggles to breathe. His eyes flicker, blinking frantically. His mouth silently gasps. The team of doctors and nurses fills the room. Chaos. I stand, unable to move. The tube is out – the thing keeping Mahesh alive. His last chance at life. My stupid mistake has killed him, or at least hastened his death.

Like all nurses, I live with too many memories, but some stand out more than others. I remember every time Mahesh blinks, every silent tear on his face, his parents' expression as they rush in and see what has happened. They are both doctors and despite being from different specialities they understand what they're seeing. Nothing is lost on them. They are looking at my face. A bad day at the office in PICU is something known only by those working there. Mahesh survives. He is skilfully and rapidly re-tubed by the Viennetta-eating consultant, a man for whom, despite our river of differences and difficulties, I have the utmost respect, even following the break-up of our twelve-year relationship, the splitting up of our family, the loss of our home. I am reminded of Mahesh, and of what my ex does regularly. He hands me slips of paper with our children's contact arrangements, on the back of which is his handover from the night before: Bed 5 DNAR (do not attempt resuscitation): not for re-intubation.

I forgive my ex his bad days, of which there are many. I know too well what is involved. I hope he forgives mine, too.

A bad day in PICU is watching a child turn purple, then black, from the outside in, and lose digits, arms or legs.

A bad day in PICU is looking at numbers from blood results and knowing they are incompatible with life; and a mother asking you if you would turn off the life-support machine if it was your child.

A bad day in PICU is caring for a child who has a brain injury so severe that a hole must be drilled in their skull to allow the excess fluid out, to notice swollen brain escaping from their head.

A bad day in PICU is caring for a child with a movement disorder, who is unable to stop moving, is jerking and constantly tense with severe muscle spasms; and knowing that these will never stop, that they are a result of contracting measles – the parents asking if the child not having the MMR meant it was their fault.

A bad day in PICU is withdrawal of care; that is, the active taking away of something that is keeping a baby alive. The removal of life. And making sense of that.

A bad day is knowing that the toddler who choked on a piece of meat at their nursery and suffered a cardiac arrest is stable now, but because their brain was starved of oxygen, it will swell over the next twenty-four to forty-eight hours and they will almost certainly be severely brain-damaged for ever, unable to walk again, or talk, or smile.

A bad day is caring for a child with Epidermolysis Bullosa, whose skin is so fragile that despite wrapping clingfilm over it, to put on a cardboard thermometer, some of the skin falls away when you touch them, no matter how gently. A layer of the child lost. A layer of the nurse lost.

A hard day at the office is cuddling a baby as he is dying, and who is alone because his new foster carer can't leave the other children, and whose birth mum's whereabouts are unknown. Stroking his head as he takes his last breath on your lap, despite you meeting him for the first time three hours ago.

It means understanding that, as tragic as PICU is, it doesn't exist in most parts of the world. The children we care for – all of them – on PICU in the UK and other Western countries simply die in other places.

For a long time after my ex and I split, I cry until my lungs can't take in enough air, my brain is fog, my skin peels off, even my bones hurt. It is my heart that is most broken. Constant chest pain, then flickering beats in my neck, numbness. My digestive system – the bowels were understood in ancient-Hebrew texts to be the seat of emotion: grief, joy and pain – leaves me feeling completely and continuously sick; I can't eat or taste or smell food. My kidneys ache, perhaps housing – as was once popularly regarded – reflection (a number of verses in the Bible state that God searches out and inspects the kidneys, or reins, of humans, together with the heart). Of course I think this to be nonsense. The digestive system, although affected by emotional experience, does not seat it. The kidneys are mechanical filters. Yet I feel sick, and then I have lower back pain for months, every time I look at my children.

'It is better that we are both separate and happy than together and unhappy,' I tell my daughter.

'No, it is not,' she says, honestly. 'Together and unhappy is better for us.'

She would rather stay in intensive care than risk living, or dying. Like the parents of a child who are contesting the doctors and nurses, in their decision to remove life support, she would rather we were alive and suffering, for the suffering of us dying is a far worse outcome for her.

Nursing becomes my life support. One of the greatest gifts that nursing has given me, aside from wonderful colleagues, and structure and job security, is the daily reminder that there is always someone worse off than you. A terrible and good gift. Time flies. Nursing changes, now I have my own children, and becomes even more intense. I have to twist my stomach into a knot, and push the image of my children away from my head, out of the PICU window, far away from the hospital.

But every night when I go home and kiss my children goodnight, no matter how much pain I feel in my heart, I am truly grateful.

Like many of my colleagues at this time, I occasionally go on retrievals to collect sick children from district general hospitals and try and help stabilise them, then bring them back to the PICU for the specialist care they need. Most hospitals do not have the ability to provide life support to very sick children. This has led to the development of specific specialist teams of retrieval (transfer) experts, able to manage the sickest children anywhere and take them to a place of safety. But at this time retrievals are in their infancy, and the team is made up of nurses and doctors who work on PICU. The coping mechanisms I am developing to deal with the extreme nature of the job are not always healthy.

I go on retrieval to a district general hospital with Dusan, and when we arrive the child is already dead. We try and try, but she is beyond any help. The first time I meet her parents is when Dusan and I have to go to a small room and tell them their daughter has died. We explain that we got there too late; there was nothing we could have done. We do not say that she went peacefully, or suffered no pain. We cannot.

On the way back to our hospital, in the ambulance, I tell Dusan that I don't feel enough. 'I should feel more about it.

Be sadder. Devastated. But I don't feel anything. Maybe I'm getting burnt-out.'

He puts his hand on my shoulder. 'We didn't know the family at all,' he says. 'Or the child. It's the job.'

But I'm worried. I went into PICU in order to be exposed to not just one speciality of nursing, but to everything: to experience the extremes of human life. To live with my eyes wide open. Instead I find I am closing down. Feeling less. Sometimes – despite horrific examples of suffering – I am feeling nothing at all.

It is noon when I finally have a piece of toast for break-fast and the red phone rings. I put my toast in the bin: there is no chance of finishing it; and I leave the coffee room, walk left down the hallways to where the red phone sits at the nurses' station, manned by one of the doctors. Trisha follows, the shadow that she has become reminding me of how I followed Anna's shadow many years before. The doctor, Ben, is taking down notes. Of course he is. Ben is one of those adrenaline-junkies who always hovers near the red phone to get the next call. Then he walks down the ward, summarising whatever he's heard: a tubed febrile convulsion in Dartford; four-year-old with meningitis; acute respiratory-distress syndrome in Southend. Incoming: respiratory failure; Stevens–Johnson syndrome; severe burns; ex-prem with AVSD (atrio-ventricular septal defect) and now pneumonia; encephalitis; malaria; sickle-cell crisis, severe chicken-pox – it is not looking good. Ben won't tell us the name of the child, just the possible diagnosis, and a judgement on how sick they might be.

At the nurses' station there is a trolley full of patient notes, which are depressingly extensive, considering the young age of the children: babies, mostly. There are computer screens and X-ray boxes showing the tiny skeletons of our patients, endotracheal breathing tubes, fragile bones, already-diseased lungs that look much too patchy, the leftover candy-floss hanging up at a funfair stall.

This phone call is about a two-year-old girl, Charlotte, in a district general hospital, who has a high temperature, a high heart rate and a few tiny purple spots of rash. It doesn't sound much. She is conscious and talking. But we understand the nature of sepsis. The hospital I work in has a speciality of treating meningococcal sepsis, a serious infection in a child's bloodstream – the most dangerous kind of infection. It can kill a child within hours. Sepsis is a disease that kills eight million people globally per year, one death every 3.5 seconds. It is an immune response triggered by an infection that has entered the bloodstream, caused by bacteria, fungus, virus or parasites. Sepsis was first described by Hippocrates as 'decay or decomposition of organic matter', and I can't think of a better explanation. The children I look after die from the outside in, their limbs like overcooked sausages, blackened, splitting open, about to burst.

It is only recently that we are allowing sepsis to have its moment: to recognise how significant a cause of death it is.

Sepsis is now understood to be the leading cause of maternal death in the UK.

Charlotte is much worse by the time the retrieval team arrives. Tracy phones me on the PICU to say they are en route back, and to get everything ready. 'She's needed so much fluid to treat her shock that her lungs are drowning in it, and she's frothing at the mouth like a rabid dog.' In sepsis, the circulating blood volume is still inside the child, but in the wrong place, extracellular – rather than intracellular. We put fluid and fluid and fluid into the veins of a patient with sepsis, in the hope that it stays there until the antibiotics start to work, but the child becomes full of fluid, blood and blood products. Charlotte needs a breathing machine to support the pulmonary oedema that we've caused, and infusions of strong medicines – adrenaline, dopamine, noradrenaline – to help her heart pump more effectively.

When Charlotte arrives on the PICU we are waiting by the door. She is on a trolley covered in tubes already, a ventilator at her head end and a monitor by her feet. Tracy hands over her details while we walk, pushing the trolley to the bed space where Dusan has rolled up his already short-sleeved shirt. Charlotte has no blood pressure at all. It is impossible to cannulate her, as her veins are too difficult to find. I position her leg in front of me – it is cold and pale, like a twig from a dying tree – and screw an intraosseous needle into her bone, confirming placement with the sudden crunch. This is a skill for which nurses and doctors practise on Crunchie bars. Trisha watches beside me, turning green. But there is no time for squeamishness. I give her a dozen easy tasks: get the fluid out, check the drug chart, run through the saline, move the bin out of the way.

We manage to resuscitate Charlotte and attach her to more machines, to take over from her failing kidneys: a more advanced ventilator called an oscillator, which she needs as her oxygen levels are so low. The oscillator makes a noise like a generator, a sort of constant chugging, and instead of effecting breaths in and out, Charlotte's chest simply shakes. Lactate is the level of acid in a person's blood and the number is a reliable prognostic factor in predicting mortality from sepsis. I write down the number of her lactate. Mortality is high (more than 46 per cent) in septic patients with both low blood pressure, like Charlotte, and lactate of more than 4 mmol/L. Charlotte has no blood pressure at all. Her lactate is 9.

The purple rash has spread. I know when I hand over, long after my shift should have ended, that it is unlikely Charlotte will be there in the morning; that she'll need three nurses at a minimum just to care for her, and she'll probably lose her almost completely dead and purple legs, and possibly her arms, too. Children as sick as Charlotte have such a profound physiological compensatory response to illness that they shut down any part of their body that is non-essential. Charlotte has kept her blood for her vital organs and has taken everything she can from her limbs. Her limbs will become necrotic. We mark Charlotte's purple-black line with a biro, to see how quickly the deadness spreads to her centre.

Adults do not do this in the same way. This will to survive – this overwhelmingly powerful and physical defiance of death – is one of the reasons I've always loved working in children's intensive care. The running towards life. Charlotte is not done yet. Her body is fighting internally as much as our machines are fighting externally. Still, we have a discussion before I leave about the lactate and necrosis in her legs and arms. 'We might need to amputate here,' one of the doctors says. 'Get the surgical team up here. It might save her, might not. But she certainly can't be moved.'

I look at the nurse taking over from me, who will likely hold Charlotte's leg as it is cut off on the ward. She is fairly junior and already this week has had to pull a mother off a child who died, the mother trying desperately to give him chest compressions after the team had stopped. She has taken another mother to the mortuary. I wonder if she still cries real tears. How much of her the job will take. Trisha has tears on her face, I notice.

What is the cost of all this to the nurses, I wonder, and how little is it valued? The surgeon will come and remove Charlotte's leg. Then leave. The amazing paediatric intensive-care doctors will spend ten minutes explaining what is happening, and why, to the family. Then leave. The nurse will hold Charlotte's leg as it is being cut off. Then she will sit with Charlotte's parents for ten or twelve hours, through the entire night, watching over Charlotte, performing her nursing tasks, as they ask her a million questions that they felt unable to ask the doctors: Is she in pain? Will she walk? Will she live? Can she hear me? Why did this happen to her? What does it mean? Do you think she will make it? Is she dying?

Charlotte should have died a hundred times over. She loses her legs and her fingertips. The extent of her illness is beyond the capabilities of our technology. Yet she survives. The neurologist Oliver Sacks wrote that 'the will to survive is stronger than disease, a miracle'. Charlotte's will to survive lifts all of us. It makes the cost worthwhile. It is easier to do the job with children like her. Easy to find the energy to be kind and to care; to prioritise, as do all nurse-parents at times, another child – a stranger – over our own.

And when Charlotte comes back to see us two years later, toddling on prosthetic limbs, smiling, looking well, holding her mum's hand and chocolates for the nurses, we all stop whatever we are doing and crowd around. Dusan walks past and stops in front of Charlotte. 'Look at you! Well, you look amazing.' His eyes meet mine. We share a look that is difficult to describe. I think of our conversations about staff morale, and of how this moment does more for the confidence in our group than anything I can think of.

Tracy comes out of the cubicle. She hugs Charlotte until she coughs. 'Naughty girl,' she says. 'Kept me so busy while you were here, and you kept misbehaving.'

Charlotte hands her the chocolates and smiles bashfully.

Tracy ruffles her hair. 'Okay, all is forgiven.'

I think of all the sunsets Charlotte will get to see. The golden skies. 'Thank you,' her parents repeat over and over again. 'Thank you.' And I suddenly feel. I feel so deeply that I have to hold my breath. I am not burnt-out yet, after all. There are more Charlottes left in my life. Charlotte is truly alive, and so am I.

9

O the Bones of the People

I keep my ideals, because in spite of everything I still believe that people are really good at heart.

Anne Frank

Of course, not every story has a happy ending. I am by now an expert nurse. But there is so much to learn, so much I still don't understand. I think about death all the time. Am surrounded by it. And don't understand why awful things happen to good people.

'If Jasmin's heart stops, she would not survive a resuscitation and, although we would do everything for her, we would not perform chest compressions in order to try and restart it.' Dusan sits next to Jasmin's aunt and has his hand on her shoulder as he speaks to her. He explains, softly and slowly, that Jasmin has suffered a lack of oxygen to her brain, a hypoxic ischaemic injury, where the oxygen levels were so low that a section of her brain has died; an injury so severe that she will most likely not wake up, and we have to let nature take its course. 'Our attempts will be futile,' he says. 'I'm so sorry.'

A nurse must judge the character of the family member. If information is given in a way that the family can't comprehend it, all manner of things may go wrong: a relative doesn't understand their loved one is dying; sometimes they can feel cheated, or tricked somehow. I am glad it is Dusan giving this poor woman the news about her niece. He is an excellent doctor. But he doesn't say the words that I can see she needs to hear. '"Do not resuscitate" is allowing a natural death to occur,' he says.

'There is nothing natural about this.' Jasmin's aunt turns to me. 'Let nature take its course?'

'She is dying,' I say.

Jasmin's aunt is too shocked to hear a narrative. She needs blunt, quick information to break through the shock. She sobs. She is crying now. She falls into Dusan, and he holds her. 'I am so sorry.' Eventually she sits up and Dusan passes her a tissue. 'Can we contact anyone for you?'

She looks at me, shakes her head. 'Can you please call the priest?'

Jasmin is a twelve-year-old girl in PICU and on a ventilator, following a house fire. Her hair smells so strongly of smoke that we are reluctant to allow her family to see her before we have tried to mask the smell. Jasmin's brother lies a few beds away, also on a ventilator but weaning off it, less sick, stronger. Their mother is dead. Jasmin is sedated and dying, but her aunt is now waiting to come in and see her. The ward's usual smell of antiseptic has been replaced with the smell of fire. Nurses cover their mouths and noses with gauze swabs. Someone asks for theatre masks. We cannot make things any better for that poor family, but smelling the lingering smoke will surely make it worse for Jasmin's aunt. Sometimes not making it worse is all we can do.

Jasmin is so sick that it is dangerous to move her at all. But I hold her head very carefully, as my colleague Nadia washes her hair as best she can, with hand-wash that she's squeezed into a gallipot, a small transparent plastic pot. That smell will stay with me for ever; it enters my nostrils and rests somewhere much deeper in my memory. As I hold Jasmin, I feel a change. Nothing changes on the monitor. Her heart rate, arterial blood pressure and SaO2 (the saturation level of oxygen in her blood) all remain the same. The ventilator does not alarm, to alert us that she may need suctioning. But Jasmin has changed; she feels lighter in my hands – something has shifted. Her head is a feather. I look up at Nadia, who is looking back at me and we both understand that Jasmin has died in that moment. We do not move for a few seconds. Take a pause. Then we both go back to the task, Nadia pulling a thick comb (her own daughter's comb, which she found at the bottom of her handbag) through Jasmin's soapy hair, tipping water gently over her. I hold Jasmin's head, letting the blackened water fall between my fingers to the plastic bucket we've put underneath. I take the bucket of blackened water to the sluice and tip it away, and the smell of smoke fills me up once more. I close my eyes and envisage the block of flats: Jasmin and her brother sharing a room, and their mum trying desperately to get to them. I hear screaming. Smell fire. I push tears back, make my stomach hard. It is not a time for me to cry.

The priest is half an hour away. There is no time to wait. I discuss what we can do, for Jasmin's aunt. She does not ask about my faith, but instead about my experience. 'Have you done it before?'

Jasmin is not the first child I have christened. We keep some holy water in the PICU in case a child is dying, the parents have not yet christened them and the priest is unlikely to make it in time. I find myself putting my fingers in the water and making a cross on Jasmin's head. If there is a God, he will surely forgive me, I tell myself.

Patients like Jasmin stay with me for ever. I carry the smell of smoke. But her story isn't the hardest part of nursing, for me. No matter how terrible, how tragic and how wrong it is, nursing teaches me that there are always worse things in life. Caring for children and adults who have been abused – as well as for their abusers – is my Achilles heel. Preserving safety is one of the main functions of a nurse. Clause 17 of the NMC Code of Professional Conduct states that nurses must 'take all reasonable steps to protect people who are vulnerable or at risk from harm, neglect or abuse'.

Hospitals have an army of staff who are primarily involved in safeguarding – protecting patients from harm.

There are child-protection nurses and doctors, safeguarding midwives, nurse specialists in domestic violence and family nurses working in the community with vulnerable younger mothers.

But it is not in the hospital that we see people who are most at risk. We walk past a lone homeless teenager at the train station. We cross the road to avoid the Romanian men sleeping under the bridge. We turn the television up when we hear our neighbours having another fight. We close our ears and our eyes to abuse – all of us.

Sky is a junior nurse and begins taking time off on a regular basis, claiming sickness, when she finds out she is pregnant. But when she returns to work she is covered in bruises that are not quite hidden beneath a thick layer of foundation, and she is breathing in sharp bursts.

'What happened?' I corner her in the coffee room.

She hooks one arm around her stomach. 'It's nothing. Did some sorting of the loft at the weekend, and I'm particularly clumsy at the moment.' She looks away, her eyes flicking back to mine, followed by a smile.

There are other signs. She never comes on nights out with other staff; but when we suggest a breakfast to say goodbye, before her maternity leave and after night duty – thinking that might be more doable – Sky is adamant that she can't make it. 'Gavin needs me at home,' she says. 'He is so protective at the moment. It's adorable.'

Gavin waits outside the hospital in the car. He controls Sky's money, giving her a spending allowance. I worry about Sky, but close my eyes and ears to it. I was clumsy when I was pregnant, I tell myself. Gavin adores her.

But three years and two babies later, Sky gets in touch and tells me about the horror of her life back then. How it started in pregnancy. How she thought Gavin would kill her.

'I'm sorry' is all I can manage. I vow not to close my eyes or ears to abuse again. And it is everywhere. Sky was right to be afraid. Domestic violence is the leading cause of death in Europe of women aged eighteen to forty-four, ahead of road-traffic accidents; ahead of cancer. I see many cases of domestic violence in my role as a nurse, and outside my role as a nurse, and three of my nurse friends have been victims.

All manner of safeguarding issues are commonplace in the NHS, as they are everywhere. Hospitals see elderly patients with fingertip bruising around the tops of their arms. Or unexplained fractured ribs; or head injuries – once a horseshoe-shaped scar on the side of an eighty-year-old man's broken cheekbone. Younger patients are also at risk. Patients with learning diffi-culties are particularly vulnerable, and those coming to the sexual-health clinic with another sexually transmitted disease. A sexual-health nurse tells me during a training day that one man is a repeat visitor, and is almost certainly being exploited. 'He won't tell us who it is, but he comes in every month with some other problem. Last month he had bite marks on his genitals. Human bite marks. He said it was his dog.'

All nurses receive safeguarding training: how to spot abuse, who to refer to and how to communicate the referral. But nurses do not routinely receive clinical supervision, as social workers do. There is no counselling for the nurse who has to swallow the stories of victims and see the physical agony of abuse. A nurse's bones become harder and more brittle with every case of cruelty she witnesses, and there are too many. My own bones are too hard.

In 2015 Greater Manchester police apologised for their failure in the case of the Rochdale child sex-abuse ring between 2008 and 2010 – failure to conduct a more thorough investigation of the allegations, and failure for some of their dealings with the victims. No officers involved faced any misconduct hearings, though Sara Rowbotham, the sexual-health nurse who raised more than 100 concerns about the victims – and whose eyes and ears were wide open – was made redundant.

Who safeguards the nurses?

I have been offered counselling twice in my career. Once, my team was offered counselling after a child's body was found by a nurse who had gone to show his parent his body, only to find it decomposing in a mortuary fridge that had stopped working. The second time was when the ECMO circuit split open and the patient's entire blood volume splattered across the walls, ceiling, staff and other patients. On both occasions, along with my colleagues, I refused. I am fairly hopeful that things are better now in nursing, and that nurses working with such extreme circumstances in areas such as critical care or A&E are offered regular clinical supervision, but colleagues tell me that no, they are not; and there's no time for it anyway.

This lack of understanding or care for nurses who are experiencing trauma is not new. After both world wars, plenty of soldiers were treated for shell shock – that is, post-traumatic stress disorder. But nurses working in the war zones were not. Research about the mental-health impact of war has always been about the men, despite hundreds of women working as nurses, next to the soldiers. In their diaries and letters these nurses describe their time in no-man's-land, suffering broken bones, amputations and gas attacks, as well as caring for soldiers with bits of their bodies blown off; the things they saw close up, the things they smelled and touched. Shell shock was never attributed to these women, and they were never diagnosed or offered treatment.

I have learned a lot during the many years of my career. Some lessons are truly painful. Others are simply shocking. Like a human skeleton, nurses must provide protection. But I learn that it's really difficult to break a child's bone, as children's bones are soft and pliable: they should not break, even with significant force. But for some children there is no skeleton, no nursing, no kindness, no protection; the damage is already done.

I learn the level of force you'd need to snap a child's leg. I learn that it doesn't take much force at all to cause a bleed in a baby's brain, just by shaking. But the baby will probably be brain-damaged so severely that the parent or caregiver who shakes that baby, unable to cope, will be even less likely to cope afterwards. I learn that prospective adoptive families do not want severely brain-damaged children. I learn, after caring for a child who was strangled by her adoptive mother, that adoption does not mean the child will always be safer. I learn to understand the abstract painting of splash marks on a child's feet and bottom, and I learn terrifying truths: 'The marks indicate that the child has been lowered into a scalding hot bath and has lifted their legs up suddenly in order to avoid the burning. But the shape of the burns on the bottom indicates they have been lowered in anyway.'

What a thing to know. The patterns of burns on a child's legs.

I find out about what was then called Munchausen syndrome by proxy (now called Fabricated or Induced Illness), where a caregiver (the mother, in 90 per cent of cases) fabricates an illness in order that her child is hospitalised, and unnecessary and sometimes painful and invasive tests are performed.

One mother I look after on a paediatric ward tricks the doctors into performing unnecessary painful procedures and surgery on her son. Every time I leave the side-room where Luke is in his cot, I leave Luke calm, content and kicking his legs. Every time I return, his mother stands over him, flinches on seeing me and Luke is screaming, the kind of cry that reaches into your bones. I stay in the room for hours, missing my break until my stomach growls, certain that the mother is hurting Luke somehow. Later the mother is diagnosed with Munchausen syndrome by proxy and she receives intensive therapy and recovers.

The hospital has a team of social workers: for child protection, mental health, older people. The child-protection social worker, along with a liaison health visitor, comes to a weekly meeting on the children's ward to discuss the cases of potential or actual abuse – those children in need or at risk, or already suffering. A school nurse sometimes comes, too. She works at various schools in inner-city London and her time is spread thin. Gone are the days where each school had their own nurse to check the children for nits and to measure weights and heights. She has been school-nursing a long time.

'I miss twisted ankles,' she says, 'and asthma pumps. School-nursing is now about gang rape, initiation to gangs by keys – that is, cutting a forearm, stabbing it really with a key, to leave a permanent scar in the shape required. It's about self-harm and anxiety disorders, prevention of online grooming by paedophiles, and drug advice. It's about sexually transmitted diseases and pregnancy. And we start that now in primary school. I have twelve-year-olds who are taking contraception. It's mostly now – like health visiting – about child protection.'

I learn the hardest safeguarding lessons during the course of my time as a children's nurse: that if you throw a toddler at the wall, or down the stairs, you can cause an injury so great that the child will suffer pain for ever – intractable seizures that never end, and a baby so stiff you can't fold them in order to change a nappy. I remember trying to fold such a baby.

Katie is only eight months old and has been on the children's ward for some time. She was born healthy. But by the time I meet her, her muscles are stiff from brain damage that she's sustained after extensive physical injuries. The doctors order nineteen X-rays of her tiny body. Her skeletal survey has revealed numerous fractures. She is considered 'failure to thrive', though she gained weight sufficiently fast with us for our conclusions to be that she has been starved. She has cigarette-burn scars all over her stomach. She is in continuous pain, despite my best efforts to calm her. I spend hours stroking her head, trying to fold her into a nappy, her hips so stiff and her legs so clamped together it is almost impossible. I weep over her, as she screams; try not to imagine what has happened to her. What her parents did. We are taught, via the media, to be afraid of strangers. That strangers hurt and abuse children. My nursing has taught me something else: it is families who abuse their children, who kill them. Parents. Caregivers. Relatives. The people we should trust the most.

Human beings are capable of such kindness. And such cruelty. A nurse has to show empathy, to remain non-judgemental, to walk in the shoes of other people. But the cruelty of child abuse fills me with horror. I cannot imagine anyone that I judge more than Katie's family. I spend many hours with them, trying to focus on my breathing. Trying to look them in the eye and not judge what they have done.

I can't help Katie.

But I do go on to adopt a child of my own.

The adoption process involves a two-day training session with social workers, whereby the kinds of children who need adoption are discussed, as well as the things that may have led the adoptees to want to adopt. But I have no language to talk about Katie, or the children and families I have cared for who have suffered.

I know more than most people in the room about why children need adoption. And the social workers are not trying to terrify the prospective adopters, but even so they reiterate that hardly any children in the UK are given up for adoption. They are, instead, removed from their birth families, due to abuse or the risk of abuse, and this can be because the birth family have serious mental-health problems, learning difficulties, drug and alcohol issues or a combination of all of these. And abuse can be sexual, emotional or physical, or neglect, or a combination of all of these. 'We are not talking about families who don't wash their children's faces in the morning,' a social worker tells me, when talking about how neglect can be the most damaging thing of all, 'we are talking about very young kids left alone for weeks, eating out of bins, eating their own vomit in some cases.'

This doesn't put me off. I have seen humanity at its best as well as its very worst and, despite all I have seen – as I'm sure all nurses agree – I believe that most people are inherently kind. The birth families who abuse their children could, most of the time, have done with being adopted themselves. I think of Mandy on the SCBU. How she is a birth mother who has abused her babies, *in utero* and post-birth, though not intentionally. How we never spoke about her own childhood, or her mother's childhood before her.

Our son comes home at eighteen months old and I carry him on my hip for six months. He is a giant baby, but he's never been my newborn. So I treat him as if he is, trying consciously to catch up on what we have both missed. I choose to funnel my care or, rather, to do everything for him so that he and I can bond, as we would have done, had he grown inside me. He feels the same way. He is physically capable of holding bottles of course, at nearly two years, but he will not. Instead he curls around me as if he is two weeks old, and I hold the bottle to his mouth, staring down at him. It is the only time he gives me eye contact. The only time he feels safe.

I feed him so many bottles, until he literally pops out of his Babygro like the Incredible Hulk: I figure that eye contact is more important than anything else at that time.

I also have a four-year-old birth daughter and a book, recently accepted for publication, with edits to look at. I am tired in a way that cannot be cured by sleep, trying to manage my baby son's trauma alongside the needs of my four-year-old. I try and continue to read to my four-year-old every night, and sometimes fall asleep with my face in *The Tiger Who Came to Tea* or *The Very Hungry Caterpillar*. Once I wake up to find it is dark and my four-year-old has closed the book I was reading and covered me with a blanket.

Despite all this, my son is not my baby for a long time. He is a stranger. We live that way for months, both of us thinking the same. He kisses me, but only through glass, crawling around to the other side of doors so that he can kiss me. There are kiss smudges all over the bottom of my glass doors. I never clean them. I remember the boy I cared for years ago, Rohan, with SCID, who was behind glass due to illness. My son has put himself behind protective glass. He is too frightened to love me.

He loves his sister, though. Immediately. And she loves him. She follows wherever he goes, a protective shadow. I find her at night stroking his head, his wide-open eyes dancing towards hers. She is gentle with him, both in physical and emotional terms: understanding that he is fragile. I am told during our training that families with birth children have a greater risk of disruption. The birth child may struggle with extreme jealousy.

Our experience is the opposite. My daughter loves him fiercely. If I say no to him, she gets angry with me. If I tell him off, she stands between us, in front of him, a protective barrier. She has endless patience, reading him the same book over and over again: a picture book of babies' faces and their emotions. I am told that children who are adopted struggle with empathy. My son feels everything that other people feel. He laughs when he sees a picture of a baby laughing. He cries when he sees a picture of a baby crying. Every time. I find my daughter ripping out the baby-crying page, and get cross with her for ripping a book. She looks at me defiantly: 'I don't ever want my brother to feel sad.'

We play a game whereby he climbs under my jumper and then out the bottom, again and again and again. He wants to be inside my tummy, born from me, almost as much as I want it. But nursing has taught me patience. Every day I keep him safe, and he keeps me safe, too. Like bones that heal slowly, we have delayed union, but I can wait. Our skeletons fuse together with kindness, understanding and play. Nursing saves me and my son from the trauma of adoption. We do not share the same blood, but we share the same bones: brittle, hard-edged and capable of healing. And, as with nursing, it is not me who saves him, but he who saves me, in the end. My hard edges soften. I feel everything intensely. He makes me a better person. A better parent. A better human.

Not every family is as lucky as we are: 20 per cent of adopted children end up returned to the care system. 'All children who need adopting have special needs,' a social worker tells me. 'They don't need normal or good enough parents, but therapeutic environments and no expectations.'

'Adoption is devastating, however you dress it up,' a friend tells me. She was adopted forty years ago. 'Helping a child is not saving a child. It is accepting that a child might not ever be saved, then loving them unconditionally anyway.'

Adoption is much like nursing: having the capacity to love a stranger.

And, like nursing, it is always sad, because every child should be able to grow up safe with his or her birth mother, and because nursing someone means that somebody is suffering in some way; but it is beautiful, too. My son grows secure and into the kindest person you will ever meet. His kindness rubs off on me. On everybody. The two things of which I am proudest in life are my son's kindness and my daughter's love for him. His relationship with his sister is more powerful than anything I have ever witnessed. My son has swallowed all the goodness of the world, and my daughter loves him like the world has never seen love. Parenting them is the greatest privilege of my life.

10

So We Beat On

Each wave breaking against the cliff would believe it was dying for the good of the sea; it would never occur to it that, like thousands of waves before and after, it had only been brought into being by the wind.

Vasily Grossman, *Life and Fate*

Cancer, like pregnancy, is invisible until it happens to you, or someone you love, then suddenly you see it everywhere. You notice the woman in the headscarf at the gym walking, not running, on the treadmill. You see the empty seat in your child's classroom, the teachers in whispers and tears. Cancer is the pollen in the air in springtime. We all breathe in the air, but only the wind controls where the pollen settles. And cancer is winning, despite our best efforts. Half of us will get cancer. Every two minutes somebody is diagnosed with cancer in the UK. All of us will be affected by it.

The oncology wards are always busy. So too are oncology outpatients and the oncology day units and chemotherapy suites. In the oncology outpatients, where patients are sometimes awaiting their first diagnosis, it is standing room only. There are lines of people leaning against the walls, too thin, sweating, in pain: a room full of people waiting to see the oncologist for a diagnosis and treatment plan, praying that the GP is wrong; and that the technician who took ages repeating the scan measurements, and not making eye contact, who said there was something a bit worrying on the scan is wrong; and that their own sixth sense is wrong. A room full of people whose entire lives are about to change for ever. A room without a floor, the patients floating in limbo, about to fall at speed; patients clutching their ticket and waiting for the flashing sign above the nurses' station to jump from number 73 to 98. The water cooler with the missing cups, and no water, empty plastic bottles lined up beside it.

The day unit is always full, and there are plenty of crash calls as patients have anaphylactic reactions to their first chemotherapy. It is a ward with no beds, but chairs that recline, and nurses flitting about between each patient to attach chemotherapy drugs to Hickman (central venous) lines, put on cold caps for the women with breast cancer who are desperately trying to save their already wispy hair, bring cups of ice to patients with terrible mouth sores, to provide relief from the treatment.

The nurses have to be extremely careful handling the cytotoxic cancer drugs. Cancer treatments were first developed during the Second World War, when nitrogen mustard gas, developed by the US army as a weapon of war, was found to cause toxic changes in bone-marrow cells. The Japanese medical community observed that the bone marrow of victims of the atomic bombings of Hiroshima and Nagasaki was completely destroyed. Sidney Farber, a Polish-American Jew, was – as was common for other Jewish people at the time – refused admission to medical school in the US. Instead he attended medical school in Germany in the mid-1920s, returning to America to study at Harvard shortly afterwards, and married Norma, a writer of children's books and a prolific poet. Shortly after the Second World War, Farber found that the drug aminopterin could treat children with acute leukaemia, by blocking a process relating to cell replication. This blocking of cell division led to modern-day chemotherapy drugs. Both Farber and his poet wife, I imagine, were searching for meaning.

Jane Cooke Wright was also searching for meaning. Her father was one of the first African-American graduates of Harvard Medical School, and after art school she followed in his footsteps and became a doctor, graduating in 1945. Jane Cooke Wright discovered methotrexate, which is a commonly used chemotherapy drug today. By her discovery she saved millions of lives. She later collaborated with Jewel Plummer Cobb, another scientist, and they further discovered that methotrexate was effective in the treatment of certain skin cancers, lung cancers and childhood leukaemia. Like both Farber and Wright, Cobb – the great-granddaughter of a freed slave – also suffered extreme racial discrimination. She was initially denied a fellowship for graduate school at New York University because of her race, although, luckily for them, and us, she was admitted after being interviewed. However, she said of her experience at Michigan: 'the popular grills and famous Pretzel Bell Tavern did not welcome black students. And so I was never allowed in the mainstream of social life on campus.'

Chemotherapy drugs are cytotoxic – that is, toxic to cells. Cancer Research UK describes chemotherapy as taking a sledgehammer to a hazelnut. Cytotoxic medication works by destroying, damaging or interrupting cellular activity at specific points in the cell cycle. But it smashes everything. In treating cancer, it can also cause cancer. The chemotherapy nurses place a 'Do Not Enter' sign on the door to the unit, ensuring that non-nurses are not taking any risks. They gown up, cover their hands with two pairs of gloves, wear masks and eye protection, ensure that nothing is broken and that everything is touched lightly, as if the chemotherapy drug itself is a newborn baby. Chemotherapy spillages are a huge cause for concern. Some chemotherapy drugs are aerobic, meaning that they can be breathed in. If the drug is spilled and inhaled or ingested or if it penetrates the skin, it may induce cancer or increase its incidence in the nurse who is handling it. This is the medicine we put directly into patients' bloodstreams. This is the reason people who are two days into treatment have legs that don't walk, and vomit bile until they are dry-retching, and even become a different colour and smell different – poisoned.

Marie Curie, a Polish migrant to France (university admission for women in Poland was forbidden), won two Nobel Prizes for her work discovering polonium and radium. Under her direction, the world's first studies into the treatment of neoplasms, using radioactive isotopes, were conducted. Radiotherapy was born. The treatment for cancer today is often a combination of chemotherapy and radiotherapy, along with surgery. Of course treatment and survival rates have increased year-on-year, due to the advancements of chemotherapy drugs, radiotherapy and to doctors' understanding of their use. We now understand the importance of careful handling of chemotherapy drugs and the dangers of radiation. Marie Curie herself developed a form of cancer called aplastic anaemia, after carrying around test tubes of radium that lit up in her lab-coat pocket like the glow-in-the-dark stars above a child's bed – beautifully chemical.

Alongside treatment, there are factors that can reduce a person's chance of getting cancer in the first place. Government health warnings advise against substances that make cancer more likely: cigarettes, alcohol, burnt toast, cleaning products, pesticides, growing up in asbestos-filled classrooms. But there are times when the doctors can find no reason as to why a person gets cancer. I've searched for meaning as to why my vegan friend who only eats organic and has never touched a cigarette or alcohol has cancer, while another friend, who lives on KFC, cider and smokes weed daily, does not. Why a friend dies in her forties as I write this book – a woman who spends her whole life helping others, leaving behind a son younger than mine. I can only remind myself, as I get older and see more and more cancer around me, to live well and happily, to value that which makes us who we are: not material possessions, but love, kindness, hope. I try to remember every day that we do not control the wind. Marie Curie's father 'enjoyed any explanation he could give us about Nature and her ways', but none of us can really explain nature. (Curie's husband slipped over during heavy rain and fell under a horse-drawn cart, fracturing his skull and dying.) Sometimes cancer cannot be explained. Or the cards we are dealt. But cancer reminds us of what matters, in the end.

I have been a nurse for twenty years. But it is only when my dad is dying, too quickly, from lung cancer, that I begin to understand the importance of kindness and the depths of humanity and philosophy underneath. When all else has failed – the chemotherapy, radiotherapy and the drugs – and hope has left the room along with the team of oncologists, radiologists, technicians and scientists, it's the nurse at his bedside who offers something else: dignity, peace, even love. Marie Curie's work did not stop after her death. About 40,000 terminally ill patients are helped by Marie Curie oncology nurses every year – those people for whom active treatment is no longer possible.

Cheryl, my dad's nurse, is performing nursing tasks with which I am, of course, familiar. She prepares the drugs that have been prescribed. After washing her hands thoroughly, putting on gloves, alcohol-wiping a plastic tray and ensuring that the area is clean in order to prevent infection, she flicks the end off a tiny glass ampoule, pushes in a needle and draws up the syrupy fluid into the syringe. Holding it vertically until the bubbles have disappeared from the bottom, she squeezes the excess air out. Ever-vigilant, she then checks the prescription and double-checks the dose. My dad's oncologist has decided on this treatment, after considering a number of scientific variables and patient-specific factors: the metabolism of drugs in relation to liver metastasis, the peak plasma concentration, the differences in the receptor-binding profiles of opioids.

She anticipates my dad's pain before it arrives, watches his body language, listens to the tone of his voice and notices the gaps in his conversation: the things unsaid. 'I'm fine,' he says. His voice is only a fraction higher than usual, but she has talked to him and has listened to him for so many hours that she knows. She administers the medication and sits next to him in silence, letting fifteen minutes pass before speaking, opening the curtains only after the pain relief has taken effect. Cheryl understands that had she not met the pain before it peaked, the medication would not have worked so well. She knows not to open the curtains until he can bear the light, and that had she done so, he'd have closed his eyes for many more hours. Cheryl understands how little time he has left, how he needs to open his eyes in order to see my mum. And how my mum needs to see him. How much peace this will give her later.

I learn then that nursing is not so much about tasks, but about how in every detail a nurse can provide comfort to a patient and a family. It is a privilege to witness people at the frailest, most significant and most extreme moments of life, and to have the capacity to love complete strangers. Nursing, like poetry, is the place where metaphorical and literal meanings cross borders. A hole in the heart is a hole in the heart; the nurse is the thing at the centre: between the surgeon's skill at fixing the literal hole, and the patient's anxiety and loss, the metaphorical hole. Nursing is – or should be – an indiscriminate act of caring, compassion and empathy. It should be a reminder of our capacity to love one another. If the way we treat our most vulnerable is a measure of our society, then the act of nursing itself is a measure of our humanity. Yet it is the most undervalued of all the professions. Anyone who works with cancer, however, understands and values nursing, perhaps knowing that it is not the cure – which so often is not possible – that matters in the end.

The Nobel Prize in Physiology or Medicine was awarded jointly in 1989 to J. Michael Bishop and Harold E. Varmus 'for their discovery of the cellular origin of retroviral oncogenes'. Varmus is a scientist who was promoted to Director of the National Cancer Institute by Barack Obama. In his Nobel Prize acceptance speech he quoted *Beowulf*, and this quote makes me think of Cheryl, of what nursing a patient with cancer is, and how important are the light and warmth of the nurse: '*Beowulf* teaches the importance of the great halls of Scandinavia during the harsh lives endured more than a thousand years ago – how the concentration of light, warmth, and vitality within those buildings offered comfort against the winter's darkness, the cold, and the constant threat of death.'

Palliative radiotherapy is like hammering a nail into a coffin with a soup spoon. A body is decomposing and is trapped in a dark coffin, but is not yet in part of the earth again. But palliative radiotherapy is sometimes used as symptom control. A tumour may be pressing on the trachea, causing a patient to choke to death, and palliative radiotherapy can target that tumour, allowing a different death to happen. A better death. Not natural, but better. The words 'natural death' are bandied around hospitals as if it's a pleasant thing to die naturally. But it is not. A natural death from cancer looks unnatural, horrific. People begin to go off, smell, rot, their veins bloated and twisted, and they sweat until they leak fluid, like cheese left in the sun after a picnic. A natural death can be the cruellest torture, and palliative radiotherapy, although also torturous, is sometimes a kinder cruelty.

My dad is dying, but now in slow motion. Still, he wants every hour, every second he can have. He is taking so much tramadol that his vision is blurry, and it is difficult for him to stay awake for long periods, but when he does, he and my mum go to the sea front and watch the waves, the light, the birds. He sees more sunsets and sunrises in the months that he is dying than he has in his sixty-three previous years. They become important. He accepts palliative radiotherapy and I am concerned. I want his eyes to fill with sunsets, and his hand to hold my mum's, and I want to smell him, my head resting on his shoulder, breathing in his jumper, and to feel the air between us – a thousand memories and the fluidity of time. I am not in my late thirties when I sit next to my dying dad. I am four again, and on his shoulders, and he is pointing at the stars, telling me about planets. I am fourteen and have broken up with my boyfriend, and he is rocking me as I sob. I am in my twenties and handing him my newborn daughter, and his face is pure joy, so total and absolute that I've never seen an expression like it, before or since. I want all of that.

On Christmas Day we go to the beach. Usually after Christmas lunch we push the planned board games to one side and fall asleep on the sofa, covered in sweet wrappers, but this is Dad's last Christmas. We know, because the chemotherapy and palliative radiotherapy and steroids are not working. We know.

The beach is cold; Dad's lips are bluish. He hates the cold. Once, he wore a jumper in the Sahara Desert, as it was 'a bit nippy out'. And here it is winter, the Irish Sea and dying bones. But I want to take a few more photographs. I try and act normal with my large camera, to sneak photographs while pretending to look for shells, to capture the colours of his eyes, which change from grey to blue to green, depending on the light.

I want to capture his colours, to have more time, and palliative radiotherapy might give me an extra day to do so, a week, maybe a month. But I don't want the spoon to hammer the nail in his coffin so slowly that he loses the spark in his eyes, that he becomes incontinent, or in pain, or leaking fluid. I've seen too much, and I can't unsee it. We do not need war and tragic road accidents to remind us of the horror of life. We have cancer.

'Jump in,' my dad pulls the cover off his bed and motions for Cheryl.

She laughs, a hearty gut-laugh, and continues to write her notes. 'You're a cheeky beggar,' she says.

Their eyes meet and smile.

It is my dad's last day on earth and, although we don't know that yet, Cheryl does. She hovers near the bedroom where he has chosen to come home to die, and only pops downstairs to make tea or phone calls or to give us space when

I'm in the room, as opposed to my mum or brother. She doesn't discuss anything nursing-related with me. Today, I am her patient's daughter. She puts her arm on my shoulder often, and sends me out of the room when she helps my dad use the commode. From the hallway, I hear them roar with laughter.

I am sitting next to him, watching Dad and Cheryl and the friendship between them, trying to understand this nursing that I've done all my life. My mum is downstairs and my brother, too. I imagine my brother holding my mum, her sobbing into him. Cheryl looks at my dad for a fraction longer than usual. I follow her eyes, though it's hard for me to look at him. My dad was never a big man, but cancer has made him small. His skin hangs off his emaciated limbs and he is a different colour, not quite yellow but sallow, his sunken eyes grey at the edges. He can't hear. He has taken the hearing aids out now and shouts everything. He can't taste. That's the worst part. 'I might as well be dead now. I can't even taste my dinner.' He looks through magazines of recipes that he will never cook: lamb tagine, cheese soufflé, Cornish turbot with bone marrow and celery, French onion soup. 'You know, I've never made *coq au vin*. Not once in my life,' he shouts.

'But you have made duck *à l'orange*,' replies Cheryl. 'With a blackberry reduction, of all things. You told me about your cooking. All those amazing things you've made.'

I tell Cheryl about our childhood, coming home to our council house in Stevenage to find pheasants that my dad had shot hanging on a door frame, or bringing a friend home for tea and finding my dad cooking stuffed hearts, or him going to the allotment every evening to pick the vegetables we'd eat that night. How my brother and I hated scrubbing mud from carrots, longed for the cleaner pesticide-ridden plastic-bag carrots we saw at our friends' houses. Dad drifts in and out of restless sleep as I talk, his funny way of sleeping with his arm in the air, hand resting on his forehead completely intact, though he jumps every time it drops. He moans. His breathing is quieter.

When I finish talking, Cheryl looks at him, then at me. 'I think we should get your mum up here, nearby.'

I don't want to nod. I don't want to acknowledge what Cheryl is implying. That Dad is so close to death. I can see his breathing is slower, and he is restless, then very still. But I'm not ready for him to go. I'm not ready.

'It's so cosy in here,' she says. 'And what a lovely day.'

The curtains are half-drawn – the light hurts my dad's eyes. But I can see the sun bathing the sky gold, a flock of birds dancing patterns in the clouds. I hear the seagull on the roof.

Dad is dying in his bed at home, with my mum holding him, my brother holding him, and me holding my mum. There is no pain. There is dignity. There is comfort. I cannot imagine a better death. We have had time to say the things we needed to, and to leave unsaid the things we didn't. My mum has time to look at him, and him to look at her. We cry, and laugh. He is totally himself until the last second. Dad is excellent at dying, it turns out. It is Mum who teaches me how to live a full life: with joy and emotion and forgiveness and truth. But my dad teaches me how to die well. He dies with humour, and dignity and a complete lack of fear. As his body shrinks, his spirit grows until the air is thick with it.

But still, I am afraid. I watch my dad's breathing get slower and more ineffective, and I want to push my mum and brother out of the way and press on his sternum, try to restart his heart, resuscitate him as I have so many others, as every muscle fibre in my body is trained to do. I can't help my dad. Today I am not a resuscitation nurse. I am not even a nurse. I am a daughter. And it hurts. Everything hurts.

I look out of the window, holding my sobbing mum as tightly as I can until she eventually gets up, and my brother holds her up. By now the sky has turned from gold to the deepest, most impossible blue. There is no moon. I rest my head on my dad's unmoving chest, listen as hard as I can for his heartbeat. But it is gone.

At night a few short days after Dad dies I am writing the last paragraph to my second novel, *Where Women are Kings*. I am under contract, in the process of editing a draft, and have been paralysed with caring for my dad, my mum, with grief. My twelve-year relationship with my children's father has irrevocably broken down. I can't imagine a darker sky. But

I want to get down what I need to say. What must be said. I don't know how things work with other novelists, but I can't separate myself from my work or my characters. I become like Elliott in *E.T.*, feeling what my protagonist feels. My characters become so real that I dream them, have conversations with them, they even argue with me. Tonight it is the other way round. My protagonist needs to feel what I feel. I will have arguments later, with my editors, about how the ending must change, and nobody will buy the book if the main character dies at the end. But my editor senses how much I need this. My first novel, *Tiny Sunbirds Far Away*, is fundamentally about survival, how some families can survive anything. But this novel is midnight. Blue-black, frightening and moonless. Some families simply cannot survive.

I return to work within days. I am numb. Cold. 'If I don't come back now, I may never be able to,' I explain to my manager, who is concerned it's too soon. But my first bleep that day is to oncology. The oncology ward is quieter than other places in the hospital. The nurses move slowly, considerately, talking in low voices. There are more visitors, flocks of families with swollen eyes huddled together outside side-rooms, coats still on. There are ten or so side-rooms on either side of a corridor, then a small nurses' station area, with various members of the multidisciplinary team rifling through impossibly large sets of notes. Pain-relief team, infection-control nurses, tissue-viability nurses, physiotherapists, bereavement nurse specialists, haematologists, oncologists, radiologists… The hospital chaplain flits in and out of rooms, offering prayer to atheists, agnostics, Muslims, Christians, people who've lived good lives and bad, regardless.

To the left of the nurses' station is another long corridor, then a main ward area, each bed separated by curtains and relatives on plastic chairs, the patients in the bed skeletal, starving, often bald, shrinking as the cancers grow bigger, attached to drip-stands and syringe-drivers delivering morphine. There is a relatives' room at the end of the corridor, where doctors and nurses give bad news. They become expert at it on this ward, understanding that honest language is the only language people understand when they are numb, and cold. 'Your husband died last night. I am sorry' is never replaced with 'passed away peacefully in his sleep'.

The nurses make phone calls, urging relatives into the hospital, while judging the likelihood that they will crash a car en route. 'Can you get here this morning? She's stable right now, but I think you should come.'

They rely on experience to tell them when the time is coming, regardless of observations or clinical blood results. They rely on a million fragments of conversations they've had with relatives, to know how to word things so that the relative gets there quickly and safely; and if they don't think it's possible, they'll call the local police to deliver the news face-to-face and bring the patient's relative to hospital quickly. On oncology wards, of all the documentation, a senior nurse once tells me, it's not the blood pressure or diagnosis or treatment plan that matters, although these are important of course. It's the relatives' phone numbers that are actually the important bit. 'Don't ever forget to write the phone numbers clearly.' There is nothing more heartbreaking than not being able to reach someone in time.

'We need to keep going with chest compressions: two more minutes,' says Ronald, a charge nurse who knows the family is two minutes away, and knows the husband well enough that he needs to be there the moment his wife dies. How important that will be. Ronald tells the junior doctor to carry on with chest compressions, despite the senior doctor's advice to stop. 'Let's do one more round,' he says. 'The husband is nearly here.'

Ronald knows that 'she is dying', even for a moment, is somehow disproportionately more comforting than 'she is dead'. He understands that the outcome cannot be changed for many of his patients, but in the small acts of kindness the outcome can be better for the relatives left behind. Illness is never about one person. The husband will not remember the doctor performing chest compressions. As the weeks and months and years fall away, he'll forget the brutality of resuscitation, the blood, the needles, the violence of pressing a body so fragile. But he'll always remember his wife's hand in his, being there when she died, whispering into her ear the words he needed to say.

I run through the ward, trying not to look at the patients too closely, but inevitably they all look like my dad in some way: the same Marks & Spencer pyjamas, the same hacking cough, the untouched fruit on the bedside table, the wife smiling too brightly. I press my teeth together as I follow the team into a side-room, where a man is sitting up in bed with an oxygen mask on his face. One of the doctors comes out, pulling off his gloves. 'False alarm,' he says. 'They thought it was anaphylaxis, but he's fine.' The team disappears one by one, but I find my feet glued to the floor. Eventually I'm alone with the patient. He pulls his oxygen mask down and smiles. 'Do you have a minute?' he asks.

'Of course.' I sit next to him and pass him the newspaper he has asked for, which is sitting next to his bed.

'Can you read the results for me?' He opens the paper to the racing results. I have a mountain of paperwork to do, and I am shortly supposed to be starting a teaching session. 'Just quickly,' he says. 'I don't want to cause a fuss, but I can't see a bloody thing without my glasses.'

I read the names of the horses and the odds.

Every now and then he punches the air. 'That's the one,' he says.

I don't look up from the paper, but I can smell the metallic odour of chemotherapy through his skin, and hear the whirring of his drip. It is the slippers, though, that do it. A pair of slippers neatly underneath the bed. Just like my dad's.

The crying that I've held in for days comes out in a rush that is so violent I knock over the glass of water next to his bed. 'I'm so sorry,' I say. 'I'm so sorry.'

I get up as if to leave, but he holds my arm. He pulls me back into the chair and then I cry. He pulls me towards his arm and tucks me there, next to his rattling chest, his ribs pressing against my cheekbones, my tears free and fast. It must have only been a few seconds, but it felt a lot longer, with him the nurse and me the patient.

'You let it out, girl.'

'I'm sorry. It's unprofessional of me. I should be helping you.'

'Nonsense,' he says. 'We should all be helping each other.'

I cry and I cry and I cry, and I wish with every cell in my body that the patient with his arm around me, who is dying of cancer, is my dad.

Cheryl is at my dad's funeral. She stands at the back, near the door, away from the friends and family, unobtrusive and respectful. Still, I can see tears on her face from where I stand at the front, holding up my mum, with my children crying beside us.

My brother thanks Cheryl as he gives a speech. 'She helped my dad die in a dignified, pain-free way, exactly as he wanted. She helped him into the hospice on the odd day when my mum really needed it. She got him there by promising whisky on the ward round. Which he got. She was at the end of the phone any time I texted her from London, day or night, and she came in on her day off when she knew it was the end. Of course she was a professional. But she was much more than that. To my family, she was our nurse. To my dad, she was his friend. She loved my dad. And my dad loved her, too.'

When it is my turn to stand up, my legs shake. I reach the lectern and try not to look at my mum, or imagine my dad's body in the coffin behind me. I'm never short of words, but today I have nothing to say. Instead I read out my dad's words – his own writing that Cheryl helped me find. She supported him to think about his funeral, decide what he wanted. She helped my mum plan, too. Told her that, officially, her plan to scatter my dad's ashes in the sea would probably need permission from someone, before my mum told her of a burly local fisherman, with a boat and no regard for the rules. 'The kind of man Ian would love,' Cheryl said.

I don't look at my mum as I read my dad's words. But I glance at Cheryl's face. I don't know how I will speak. My voice is choked. But her tiniest of nods gives me the strength to hold the piece of paper up, stand straighter and read:

'Love is the only thing that matters. I'm talking about you and me, here: the love that you share with your wife, or

husband, or lover, and your son and daughter, and then –
perhaps the most precious love of all – with your grandchild.
I'm talking about a love so deep you'd give up your life to
defend it. A love so high you can glimpse heaven, enough to
believe in it. Maybe some of you have seen it already. Maybe
some of you are as lucky as I am. That's all I have to say. Fall
in love. That's the only thing that matters, in the end. Love
each other.'

11

At Close of Day

The true measure of any society can be found in how it treats its most vulnerable members.

Mahatma Gandhi

Dying is not always the worst thing. Living a long life and suffering cruelty in old age is the terrible fate that waits for many of us. We will all get sick and die, or we will get old. We can only hope that those caring for us are kind, and that they are empathetic and altruistic. But can these traits be learned? Are they inherent or changeable?

Since Darwin argued that morality pre-existed religion, altruism has been studied by scientists, theologians, mathematicians, evolutionists and even politicians, but the origins of kindness remain a mystery. Darwin himself acknowledged the idea that survival of the fittest perhaps encompassed survival of the kindest. For any civilisation to be fit, and to survive, its members had to be collectively kind – to make personal sacrifices for the greater good of the group. George R. Price, a science journalist, further discovered an equation that proved that selflessness was part of a larger survival tapestry; that altruism is not selfless and moral, but rather selfish and genetic. He could not cope with this thought. He wanted to believe that we are fundamentally kind, that we are good. Price spent the rest of his life performing acts of social justice and random acts of kindness, before eventually killing himself, cutting open an artery, much as Derek had tried to. He could not make sense of this world.

I struggle to make sense of anything, but at last I know what nursing is. I learn the lesson the hardest way of all. I watch Cheryl like a hawk, with the same intensity I watched the first nurses I ever saw, all those years ago. And this time it is personal. It takes being on the other side of the fence for me to really understand the importance of kindness. It takes my dad dying for me to understand how precious and fragile and vulnerable we all are – not just the patients in hospital, but all of us; and that our own day will surely come when we have to rely on the kindness of strangers. It is the realisation that my dad will be your dad, maybe already has been. That you and I will be Gladys or Derek or Jasmin's aunt. Nursing is simpler than I thought. It doesn't really need theorising. Nursing is helping someone who needs help.

But of course, as in all sections of society, we know that some nurses are not kind. Many of the misconduct cases against nurses that were listed on the Nursing & Midwifery Council website were related to care of the elderly: shocking examples of bad nursing care; cruelty; patients who were physically hurt or restrained by nurses, shouted at, sworn at, kicked and punched.

Care of the elderly is the truest form of nursing there is. In nursing older people, technology becomes a lot less important. Medicine becomes less important. Even cure. What matters is the heart of nursing: dignity, support, care, tenderness and respect. But we have a crisis. The number of older people in England is increasing more quickly than we can cope with, and the Department of Health predicts an increase of 20 per cent over the next decade. As our population gets older, this area of the hospital is bursting at the seams and, with cuts to social care, there is often nowhere to send a medically fit elderly person who needs basic nursing care, and so they stay in hospital, taking up the bed of another patient who might need it medically. The NHS spends £820 million a year on keeping older patients in hospital when they no longer need acute treatment. There is inadequate funding in community healthcare, and the health system is buckling under this pressure. Older people in hospital deteriorate quickly; for example, they lose 5 per cent of muscle strength for every day of treatment in a hospital bed. The longer their discharge is delayed, the less likely it is that they will be discharged and the more fragile people become.

Care of elderly people in hospital is changing. Hospitals are becoming a place where older people are having complicated surgeries, with a view to preserving or enhancing their quality of life. 'Do Not Attempt Resuscitation' forms are still common on care-of-the-elderly wards, but it is rare now (as used to be commonplace) for doctors to write in the reason box: 'elderly, frail, would likely be futile'. Instead, unless a patient has advanced cancer, end-stage renal failure or heart failure, they are given the same capacity to experience quality of life whether they are sixty-five or ninety-five, and hospitals are performing riskier and more complex treatments on older populations.

This cultural shift as we age has significant implications for any health system. Nursing older people is heavy work: hoisting incontinent patients into a chair to change the bed, chatting all the while; washing, toileting, dressing, cleaning dentures, brushing hair, helping to hold a spoon or cup, puffing up pillows or holding hands. Many older people have a long hospital stay, are sent home inappropriately early and without the care they need, only to bounce back to hospital in an even worse condition. The nurses run between patients, performing a constant stream of tasks: a conveyor belt of washing, drugs rounds, turning, changing beds, serving meals that you would not serve to a dog, and occasionally (as one nurse did often) smuggling in home-cooked lasagne. The drugs round takes for ever. The staffing levels are often unsafe, despite the government statement following the Francis Report that 'Older people should be properly valued and listened to, and treated with compassion, dignity and respect at all times.'

Most of the nurses I've ever worked with are kind, compassionate and caring. But, as with any job, even a good nurse can have a bad day. It may be influenced by what is going on in her personal life, but also by external and political pressures. It is hard to be kind when you are undervalued by society, by your employers and by the media. It is hard to always be kind when you are exhausted and working continually in an unsafe environment. Burnout – that is, long-term unresolvable workplace stress – is common and serious: research has shown it can cause mental-health problems as well as coronary heart disease. And there is another risk for nurses, sometimes known as secondary traumatic stress disorder, or compassion fatigue. Compassion fatigue was first diagnosed in nurses in 1950 and can cause sufferers constant stress and anxiety, as well as having a terrible impact on their ability to provide the quality care, kindness and compassion that patients need and deserve. In one study up to 85 per cent of emergency-room nurses were suffering from compassion fatigue. This is different from burnout, which is a long, slow process and is shown to be a kind of depression. Compassion fatigue is common when caring for people who have suffered trauma. The nurse repeatedly swallows a fragment of the trauma – like a nurse who is looking after an infectious patient, putting herself at risk of infection. Caring for negative emotions puts her at risk of feeling them, too. And taking in even a small part of tragedy and grief, and loneliness and sadness, on a daily basis over a career is dangerous and it is exhausting.

But there is no excuse for bad nursing care. None. I am horrified if ever I see a bad nurse. I am thankful I've only seen bad nurses a handful of times during my career, and the vast majority of nurses are kind, compassionate and caring in all circumstances. And luckily, kindness is also contagious. But I have seen plenty of good nurses have bad days. And there is a much wider political context to examine. On a care-of-the-elderly ward there can be thirty beds and two qualified nurses.

The staffing levels are so bad this week that the nurses, the ward sister tells me later, often don't take a single break the entire day. A nurse I know who works on the ward carries glucose tablets in her pocket, in case her blood sugar drops dangerously low: she has fainted at work a few times on days when there hasn't been enough time for lunch or dinner breaks. Another nurse has repeated cystitis and has been told it was because she didn't go to the toilet when she needed to. There are times when you literally don't have time to go to the toilet; days when you purposefully don't drink water, as you know you won't have time.

Of course the world is shifting: there is something deeper in our society alongside appalling staffing levels. We are separatist, disconnected from each other and our social values are changing. We glorify youth. Older people are not considered – as they are, for example, in West Africa and other parts of the world – wise and important members of the community. Our elderly are considered burdens. We dread ageing. And rightly so. Although older people contribute £61 billion to the economy, according to Age UK, nearly 900,000 older people now have unmet needs for social care.

I feel as if I have no kindness in me at the moment. I am exhausted. I have split from my children's dad, we had to sell our house and I can barely afford my rent. I'm working ridiculous hours, nursing and writing and teaching, and even that is not enough. I am not one of the many nurses who has taken a pay-day loan or gone to a food bank, but I am dangerously close. I find my daughter putting Sellotape in her shoes. She jumps when she sees me, tries to hide the shoe behind her back. When I see the school shoes and the massive holes in them, she puts her arm around me. 'It's okay, Mum,' she says, 'because when it rains, the rain doesn't go in the holes any more.' She is ten years old.

I am a failure. I feel like the worst mother alive.

I miss my dad.

I finally know and understand what nursing is, I have the skill and experience to be an expert nurse, but I am not sure I have any energy. I am depressed, burnt-out and tired. I certainly feel as if I have compassion fatigue.

You can often smell the care-of-the-elderly wards from the outside. Incontinence is common and, with staffing frequently at dangerously low levels, washing, toileting and dignity are the first things to fall away when there is a medical emergency. I walk through the smell, which is bad enough to make my eyes water, towards the group of people surrounding a bed, a doctor on the bed itself performing chest compressions on a man so small you can hear cracking ribs. A crunching sound, like walking in fresh snow. There are enough people surrounding the bed, and the chances are most of them do not need to be here.

Instead I go to answer one of the many flashing call bells, to another man who is clearly in pain. Walking past the patients on a care-of-the-elderly ward is a lesson in living well. The Book of Job describes human life as inherently limited. But we go on after our bodies stop. All the patients on the care-of-the-elderly ward look semi-decomposed, as if they are falling back into the earth. The beds seem to swallow some of the people whole. There are older patients throughout the hospital: on the medical and surgical wards, in the outpatient departments, oncology, the mental-health unit. But a care-of-the-elderly ward is where you see the very, very old and incredibly frail. Where the patients might be recovering from falls at home, or confused, suffering from repeated chest infections. On either side of me four bedded bay areas house impossibly old men. The women's section is across the corridor.

A man with paper-thin skin and concave cheeks is pushing a shaky hand towards his tray, where tea in a thick plastic adult sippy cup, which has teeth-shaped marks on the spout, has been set slightly out of his reach. He doesn't, or can't, speak. His information is written above his head on a large whiteboard, in terrible handwriting. There is a similar board above the nurses' station that reads: 'Remember: Speak English'.

The patient's board is written in green pen: 'Mr Guilder. No allergies.' On the board is written 'Visiting Time: 3–5 p.m.', but there's no evidence of visitors, with him or anywhere else on the ward. The lack of family members coming to visit elderly relatives is a source of astonishment for my international colleagues. 'You don't see this in other countries. Elderly people with nobody next to them. Living alone. Being cared for by strangers.'

I stop, take a breath and try and find some energy to help. My eyes are barely open, watering because I'm so exhausted. But I can't walk past. The nurses on the ward are too busy, and nobody is in sight, although I can see an open cubicle door and dirty linen in bright-yellow bags being thrown out in a pile.

I look at my watch. I can't be late to pick up my son and daughter from childcare. I imagine them sitting, the last children in the after-school club, as they always are, their faces staring out of the window until they light up when I arrive. 'I'm sorry,' I say. 'Don't worry, Mummy,' is always the reply. They never ever complain. Which makes me feel worse.

But then I look at the man in the bed, his expression, his loneliness.

I flash back to my mum after long days as a social-work student and weekend work in a factory to fund the studies, her volunteering night shifts for the Samaritans. She must have been exhausted, but somehow she was always kind. I think of Cheryl, and of how much she meant to my dad, how much she was there – often on days off, her own life taking second priority to the kindness that my dad so desperately needed.

'Hello, Mr Guilder,' I say, half-pulling the curtain between him and the chaos of the ward, the rushing staff and call-bell alarms. I sit on the chair next to his bed, without giving too much thought to the wetness on the seat. I reach for the lukewarm tea and hold it in front of him. His hand shakes violently. 'Let me help you.' I support his head with one hand and tip the cup towards his dry, cracked lips. He drinks like a man who has been unimaginably thirsty. I don't let myself think about when he last had a drink. It isn't necessarily the nurses' fault. There are no staff today. But none of that helps Mr Guilder. His face becomes less twisted as he drinks, his shaking subsides. After the tea's finished, he leans back in his bed, exhausted from the effort of simply staying alive. He smiles and is a fraction more peaceful.

He's shivering, though. The blanket that covers him is almost as thin as his paper skin. 'I'll get you another,' I tell him. 'It's cold today.'

I walk past the locked drugs cupboards, past the double sinks and the large whiteboards containing patient lists, consultant names and a large section where the nurses are now required to write: 'Number of Falls in Last Month', 'Number of MRSA Cases Last Month', 'Number of Pressure Sores', and other preventable horrors that should not happen in hospitals, but frequently do. I walk past the patient toilet to the linen cage, where there are sheets and pillowcases, but no blankets. The nurse in charge walks past in a hurry. 'There's no delivery until later. I've phoned them already. You'll need to borrow one from another ward.'

Along the corridor is the private patients' ward, ever-expanding. It is another world. They seem to have everything and never run out. My team has been auditing the cardiac-arrest trolleys to check they have everything they need, and nothing extra (too many boxes of gloves; banned, old-type nasopharyngeal tubes; old batteries; out-of-date defibrillator pads; and, once, a jewellery box filled with buttons). There is, or should be, a hypoglycaemia kit attached to the trolley in case the patient's blood sugar drops dangerously low, and containing, among other things, a bottle of Lucozade. Many times that is missing, and the nurses often blame junior doctors on their night shifts – in need of energy after twelve hours on their feet.

Unlike the ward next door, entrance to the private patients' ward is by entry-code only. These units in NHS hospitals are ever-growing, and sometimes NHS patients are sent to private units as there simply is no NHS bed. This is damaging to the NHS. Tife, the site nurse practitioner, once commented: 'If you do something in plain sight, nobody realises. Privatisation is happening right in front of our eyes.'

I buzz and wait until the receptionist lets me in with a bright voice. I walk along the spotless corridor, past the patients' relatives, mostly Middle Eastern men wearing designer trousers and sliders. Of course many patients choose to stay at home, often being cared for by Western nurses and doctors in the Middle East. Plenty of nurses have worked in places like Saudi Arabia, spending a year or two making money there, to clear debt or save for a small deposit for a flat back home. You can earn better money, most of which is tax-free, and live in a place where you have minimal costs. I could never do it. On returning, a friend told me, 'As a female nurse, you get ignored by the men, disrespected and not listened to. Sometimes spat on. It's a complicated business, gender and culture in other parts of the world. You learn a lot, and not all of it good.'

My doctor friend Mohammed is from Oman, and gives a different view of nursing and medicine in the Middle East. 'Things are changing. Attitudes to women are improving. People have respect for nurses. The money is good, but the heat is awful. I'm happier here in the English rain.' He collects umbrellas of every colour and size and, instead of a photo of his smiling face on the welcome board, there is his name and a photograph of a yellow umbrella.

In the private patients' ward every patient gets their own room, with an en-suite bathroom and a television. All is immaculate, clean, with a desk area, a comfortable chair and a large mirror. On the table next to the bed is a menu with numerous options for meals, including kosher and halal, and there is an Arabic version on the back. Next to the menu is a small transparent packet of Molton Brown toiletries and some fluffy slippers wrapped in plastic. The beds have extra blankets and there are two pillows, in immaculate soft white pillowcases. If it wasn't for the oxygen and suction, you could be in a five-star hotel. I take a few minutes of quiet to look out of the window, think about the old plastic cup of luke-warm tea slightly out of reach of the elderly patients next door. I find the linen cupboard and, with nobody around, help myself to two blankets and tuck them underneath my arm for Mr Guilder.

When I get back, the hospital hairdresser is brushing a man's hair in the bed next to him. I smile at them. What an important job. Skin-hunger is something that we talk about – the lack of physical contact that older people might have with others. Imagine never being touched. Studies have shown that positive physical contact, such as hugs, are associated with measurable and meaningful attenuation of blood pressure and heart rates in adults.

Mr Guilder is asleep. He looks almost dead, all open-mouthed and gasping, but elderly people can sleep that way.

I leave him and walk over to the women's section to a patient called Mrs Jones, who reminds me of many of the women in my own family: particularly my maternal nan, who is also a straight-talking Welsh woman with perfectly curled hair, whose eyes fizz with humour. And, like many of the women in my family, Mrs Jones is a real character, very old and extremely tough. She has Chronic Obstructive Pulmonary Disease (COPD) and needs oxygen around the clock in order to breathe. Her lungs have left her immobile, and her muscles have wasted to the extent that she can no longer walk and relies on a wheelchair. She also has a host of other health disorders, including heart failure and diabetes, but that doesn't stop her enjoying life. She's ninety-two and can finish a difficult crossword puzzle in seconds.

'Slip me some extra insulin this evening, Nurse,' Mrs Jones says to me, smiling. 'I've been a bit irresponsible.'

I stop and look through her notes. She had a crash call last night, but no cardiac arrest. 'Been on the gin again, Mrs Jones?'

Mrs Jones suddenly laughs. Giggles. Puts her hand over her mouth. Her age melts away and she looks twenty years old. 'I've got a few things,' she says. 'Brought in to me.' Patients smuggle all manner of things into hospital: booze, drugs, Avon products to sell to other patients. Worse, patients and relatives take things out of hospital, too: nurses' handbags, drugs, televisions, other patients' contraband, even a six-foot grandfather clock. The replacement grandfather clock is now chained to the ground. 'There is nothing more sad,' says my colleague, 'than seeing things chained up in an NHS hospital, in case someone nicks them.' But theft is commonplace. At Christmas time all the presents left by a charity at a hospital, for the children fighting for their lives in intensive care, are stolen. One night a nurse's purse is stolen from her bag lying next to her head, while she is taking a sleep break. Nurses are careful not to take cash to work, and always to make sure their bags are locked in an office, lest someone steals money from their purses while they're working.

'No, even worse than gin,' says Mrs Jones. 'Häagen-Dazs.'

I raise my eyebrows. A healthcare assistant had told me earlier, 'Apparently she always has a cupboard full of sweet things. We never get to the bottom of where she sources the sweets and chocolates from, but I suspect one of the other patients who has been known to climb into the wrong bed, and in with other patients.'

But ice-cream? That's impressive. Aside from smuggling in contraband, Mrs Jones is able to make the other patients laugh. She's always cheerful, despite the pain that I know she must have, with the exacerbation of her COPD, but suddenly she stops smiling. I see a group of people coming towards us.

Dr Robertson is performing a ward round. As with the nurses, occasionally a doctor is not kind. And Dr Robertson is universally hated by patients and staff alike. He postures around the ward, barking orders to anyone nearby (he once asked the cleaner for his patient's blood results, and was furious when she told him she was there to make the afternoon tea: 'Well, can't you find out? Or find someone who can?'). He has the worst bedside manner of anyone I've ever worked with. And that includes the surgeon who throws things, and the consultant who smiles every time she gives a patient bad news. But the vast majority of consultants I've ever worked with are kind, exceptional and often eccentric.

But Dr Robertson is not merely eccentric, he is unkind. We spend many hours thinking up things that might upset him, tricks we might play on him to give us some sense of fairness. But it's not only Dr Robertson who is disrespectful and unkind to patients.

'Mrs Jones is a ninety-two-year-old woman suffering extensive co-morbidities and COPD. We'll examine her, and you can all give me her differentials,' Dr Robertson says to the medical students hovering around him, but not once does he glance at Mrs Jones.

Jayne, the nurse on the ward round, is scowling. The medical students are a mixture of serious-looking young Indian men and white women wearing high heels. It seems to be that the female medical students frequently wear pencil skirts, low-cut tops and heels to work. I have no idea why. A few years of being covered in body fluids and running through hospitals will probably encourage flat shoes and less expensive-looking clothing.

'Mrs Jones, we are going to examine you,' Jayne shouts. 'Sit up properly for us. There's a good girl.'

I close my eyes. I'm surprised Mrs Jones doesn't swing for her. When I open my eyes, though, she's smiling. 'What's that, love?'

'It's Dr Robertson,' Jayne shouts. 'He's going to examine you now, dear.' She shouts at the top of her lungs. Mrs Jones pulls her ear down. Cups her hand around her earlobe. Jayne leans close. The medical students lean closer behind her, as if glued to an invisible thread. 'Doctor will examine you, dear. Make you better.'

After a few minutes of Jayne shouting loudly enough to bring the healthcare assistants from the office, the patient in the next bed begins tutting and then starts her own shouting. 'No rest, no rest.'

Mrs Jones lets her hand drop. 'I'm not fucking deaf,' she says. 'And you can't fix me, dear. I'm not fucking stupid, either.'

They scramble away in a group, Jayne looking red-faced. Unfortunately, this is not the only time I've witnessed nurses who are patronising, dismissive, unsympathetic and sometimes simply cruel to patients. There is a nurse I work with who, frankly, I wouldn't let look after a hamster. She is rough with all the patients, makes huffing noises when asked to do anything, and sits at the nurses' station flicking through magazines while the call bells flash red above her. Her patients suffer as a result. Become sicker, even. Or at least don't get better so quickly. As Florence Nightingale observed: 'If a patient is cold, if a patient is feverish, if a patient is faint, if he is sick after taking food, if he has a bed-sore, it is generally the fault not of the disease, but of the nursing.'

I wonder whether it's getting worse, and whether doctors and nurses are becoming less kind to patients, or whether we have rose-tinted glasses for the good old days of nursing. I wonder if our society is suffering a collective form of compassion fatigue. *Hiraeth* is a Welsh word for nostalgia, or a longing for something you can never return to or that never was. I hope we can return to kindness, if it existed. And if not, I hope we can all be like Mrs Jones. Let us rage against the dying of the light.

12

There Are Always Two Deaths

There must be another life, here and now... This is too short,
too broken. We know nothing, even about ourselves.

Virginia Woolf

Hildegard Peplau, a prolific writer and academic nursing theorist, wrote that the final stage of a nurse–client relationship (which lies at the heart of what nursing means) is one of resolution and termination. The nurse and client only end their relationship if a patient is discharged or dies. 'One of the key aspects of a nurse–client relationship, as opposed to a social relationship, is that it is temporary,' Peplau said.

She was wrong. Nursing does not stop when a shift at the hospital ends. And it does not stop after death.

A tiny white coffin: the funeral of another baby. The baby that my nursing colleagues and I cared for over the course of six months on PICU. Samuel was born too soon, his lungs underdeveloped, and required so much ventilatory support that he developed chronic lung disease: a condition that makes the lungs stiff, difficult to oxygenate and prone to infections that are severe enough to require life-support machines. Every winter PICUs are full to breaking point, full of Samuels, former premature babies who survived at twenty-three or twenty-four weeks and were not the lucky ones who went on to develop normally. Nurses understand the dangerous end of developmental uncertainty: that families have often been through countless traumas following an early birth, only to end up on paediatric intensive care a year on, their now even more beloved child fighting for survival again.

Samuel's mother's face is permanently twisted in agony, her eyes searching, but not seeing. The funeral is well attended, with family members all gathered in their pain, their faces soaked with tears. I look around the church at the mourners. We all love Samuel. I count six nurses, including me; three of them travelled for two hours, following a night shift, and have now been awake for twenty-one hours.

One nurse, Jo, looked after Samuel the most. Jo is a junior nurse on PICU and, as Samuel had a hospital-acquired infection, he needed caring for in a side-room, away from the rest of the ward. Jo spent the last few months in that room: twelve-and-a-half-hour days sitting beside Samuel and his mum; twelve-and-a-half-hour nights alone with Samuel, while his mum slept in nearby parents' accommodation. I'd go into the room occasionally to relieve Jo for a quick break, or to check a drug with her, and she would be singing to Samuel, or holding his hand, or stroking his hair. His eyes followed her around the room, and he smiled at her as if he really meant it, even though he must have been in pain. Jo kept bubbles in her pocket and blew them gently above him, popping them one by one until Samuel kicked his legs. When a consultant gave bad news to his mum, Jo was there, and stayed long after her shift to translate into plain language what he meant. When it was time for Samuel to die, Jo painted his hands, made prints on a card. She took a curl from the back of his head and gave it to his mum.

To give that much of oneself is dangerous. Grief can only be swallowed so many times before it damages. There is too little clinical supervision for the weight of emotion that nurses feel, and the things they see or do are so little explored, in terms of how it may or may not affect their own lives. Good nurses, though, will risk the danger and hurt in order to help. Jo was bent in half during the service, and afterwards I watched Samuel's mum approach her and they held each other in the middle of the church, while the grief that filled the air clouded the tiny white coffin beside them.

The NMC Code of Professional Conduct states:

20.6 Stay objective and have clear professional boundaries at all times with people in your care (including those who have been in your care in the past), their families and carers.

But there is no objectivity in good nursing care. Jo was a brilliant nurse. She understood that to nurse is to love. Even after death.

*

The 'last offices' – that is, the care given to a person after death – is a nursing task. Laying out a body is the most intimate thing you can do for another human. It is a secretive process, like much of how we deal with death in the UK, and something you cannot really learn in a classroom.

The first dead body I see is on a general medical ward. I am in training and on placement. The nurses I work with are smokers (one of them is heavily pregnant and is still popping out for cigarettes) with too much jewellery and bad haircuts. The patients on this ward suffer from all manner of medical problems – diabetes and dementia, heart failure and chronic lung disease, leg ulcers and broken hips – and need help with eating, drinking, toileting. The cycle of work is one of repetition. We wash people in succession, based not on whether they have urgent needs to use the commode, but on bed numbers: bed one washed and up first. If the patient in bed one is asleep, they are woken.

But today everything is late. The patients sit up in bed, looking happy that they are not being made to sit on a chair or walk up and down the ward.

When I go into the side-room, two of the nurses are massaging a dead man's joints. I am pushing a tea trolley. The trolley shakes, makes a clanging noise. I stop and stare, and don't realise that my mouth has dropped open until one of the nurses, Kelly, looks up. 'Aw, love, don't worry. He had a good life and was comfortable. Family all came at the end.'

'I'm sorry,' I say, backing up with the trolley. 'I haven't seen it before.'

I walk slowly backwards, almost bowing with every step, sensing the need for formality and reverence. I notice how both nurses massage his hands and wrists as if he is alive, though it is clear he is dead. His skin is completely grey, his mouth open, and he does not look human.

'Leave the trolley out, and you can give us a hand,' says Kelly.

I want to say no. I want to make an excuse and never see a grey dead person again. But I know I need to be tough.

I take a breath outside the door and then go back in, minus the trolley, wearing an apron. 'You can start with the elbows,' Kelly says. 'Rigor mortis already, but we can massage it away.'

I feel sick in my mouth and swallow hard. I try not to think about the man in front of me as a person: it's the only way I can get through it. I think simply of his elbow, by now the colour of miso soup, as I rub it gently, trying to make it less stiff: to make him less dead. I try not to look at the photograph of the children. Grandchildren? Great-grandchildren?

Kelly eventually explains what they are doing – massaging the rigor mortis, before propping his arms up with a pillow, 'So that his arms don't get discoloured or pool,' she says. 'Nothing worse than pooling, for the family. Then we put his teeth in and prop his jaw with a pillow. Then we wash him. Spruce him up a bit. And label him, then wrap him in the sheet. We need to do this in summer. If a fly gets into his nose or mouth, there'll be maggots pretty quickly. Nothing more terrifying for the family.'

I focus on the other nurse, who is pregnant and muttering, 'Shroud, not sheet.' I do not dare ask what 'pooling' is. I focus on trying to remove the image from my head of a body infested with maggots, of flies climbing inside us after we die, of the horror of our humanity.

Later that day I take a walk outside during my lunch break at around 4 p.m.

'Penny for them,' says a man on the bench next to me.

'Life and fate,' I say.

He laughs. 'That sounds serious.' He turns his face towards the sun, closes his eyes. 'What a beautiful day.'

I have Savi with me, a junior nurse. We are preparing the body of a six-year-old who has drowned in her grandparents' pond. The room is too bright, despite our efforts to make sure the blinds cover each section of the window.

The room is bathed in mustard light. The girl at the centre of it, Freya, is too small in the bed, her head still resting on a pillow, her eyes half-open, despite our best efforts. I keep gently resting my fingertips on her eyelids, trying to close them. But they spring open as if she is waking from a terrible dream. The parents and grandparents and two older siblings – eight and ten years, respectively – have chosen not to be in the room while we perform these last rites. They wait in the family room near the ward entrance, and I try not to imagine them in that room: what they can't say to each other, and how the grandparents, particularly, must feel. Every death is a little tragedy, but Freya's death is cruel.

She has a catheter, an ET tube, a CVP line, two peripheral cannulas, an intraosseous needle still inserted in her bone, a chest drain, a nasogastric tube. 'We can't take everything out,' I say to Savi. 'We need to leave everything in and bung it, or pack it. I'll cut the ET tube just inside her mouth and pack around it, so it doesn't look too bad. It's very upsetting for the family, of course.'

Savi is standing behind me, although the large room is now devoid of machines and there is space surrounding the bed. 'It's the first dead body I've seen,' she says.

I take a breath. I always forget. Now that I am older and have been doing the job for so many years, I have lost touch with my younger self and the extent of my emotion. I wonder if I feel as much. There are always people other than the family who are devastated by the death of a patient in hospital: the doctors, the nurses, the lady who brought tea and biscuits and chatted to the patient every day, the healthcare assistant who helped the patient read the menu, the hairdresser who came to the ward, the pharmacy assistant who checked the drugs chart and stopped to chat a while. But it's the junior nurses who tend to feel the most; the senior nurses have found ways to turn their hearts into ice, in order to enable self-preservation. But developing that level of thick skin takes years of practice. I cannot count exactly how many dead bodies I've seen, but there have been too many. Nurses spend a long time with dying patients – those between worlds, between words – and with those recently dead, when they are not yet mortuary-dead and their lungs still contain air, the room still holds the smell of their nightdress and the sound of their voice. Particles of them float; dust in the light.

'Sometimes it helps if you talk. Out loud, I mean,' I say to Savi. 'As if the child is still here.'

Savi comes out from behind me. She has a face full of tears. 'That poor family,' she says.

I reach my arm across her and hug her gently. 'It's okay to cry. Good, actually. It shows the family you really care.' I will my own tears to come, but they are too deeply buried inside me. 'Cry,' I tell my dry eyes. 'Cry!'

'In my culture you have limited time to cry. Hindus believe that mourning should take place for thirteen days. It's also the family who wash their loved ones. Not the nurses.'

'It sometimes is here,' I say. 'But not always. It's best to ask the question and support whatever the family wants. The parents are in so much shock they can barely stand up...' I look at Freya. Her body is bloated, bruised and grey, covered in equipment. 'Let's get to work,' I say to Savi. And then to Freya, 'Okay, sweetheart, we're going to give you a little wash.'

Like many of my colleagues, I always talk to dead people. It makes them somehow less dead, allowing nurses to perform the things they have to do without breaking down in grief, or feeling their own mortality biting the air. Talking to dead people keeps them alive. There is an atmosphere in the room after a person has died, which you can sense if you have felt it before, like an argument – something hanging in the air. Most of the nurses I know are pragmatic and practical, and believe that dead bodies are just that. We are all simply dust, dancing in the air. But of course every nurse has a ghost story.

'You fill up the water, and I'll begin.'

Savi fills a bowl with warm water.

'Make it hot,' I say. 'It will keep Freya from being too cold, when the parents come in.'

Savi sniffs and looks away.

'Take your time,' I add. My face is so dry it itches.

I clean down a plastic tray with an alcohol wipe – habit more than anything else: Freya is not now going to develop infections. But these habits keep things normal, as if I'm touching a central venous pressure line from a living child. There is no blood, but there is fluid leaking from her tissues around the edges of things. I try and cover as much of it as possible with gauze. I undo the tapes and put fresh dressings on her skin, over the tubes. She is pooling fluid underneath her arms, too. I move them, massage them slowly, to make them seem more normal when the parents come in. I know what pooling is now. All too well. Secret words like 'hypostasis' are no longer strange to me.

Savi begins to wash Freya's skin; she takes her time and is gentle. She is humming. When she has washed Freya from top to toe, she puts her hand on Freya's chest. 'Lead us from untruth to truth,' she says, 'from darkness to light.'

'You look much better,' I say to Freya, as her eyes finally stay closed. And she does. Her skin shines with the baby lotion that Savi massaged onto her after the wash, and she is now dressed in pyjamas. Freya looks less dead, more asleep. 'Final thing,' I say. I rummage in her bedside drawer and find a small toothbrush with a pink dinosaur head-cover. I snap it open, and put a pea-sized amount of Freya's bubble-gum toothpaste onto the brush, before brushing her small, square and perfectly white teeth until I smell nothing but bubble gum.

In the NHS the staff completely reflect the patients they serve: the nurses, doctors, porters, healthcare assistants, catering staff, cleaners and technicians come from all corners of the world – every background, race, culture and religion possible. I have worked with nurses who are atheist, Buddhist, evangelical Christian, Muslim, Sikh and Catholic; nurses who were nuns, as well as those who belong to religions I've never heard of. 'I believe in crystal-healing and angels,' a nurse colleague once told me. 'My religion is vodka,' said another. But whatever my colleagues believe, and no matter how dormant or non-practising their faith is, the nurses' own beliefs become important when a patient dies.

From its earliest days, Christianity encouraged its devotees to attend to the sick. But from the earliest times many cultures produced nurses who were dedicated to service on religious principles. Many nurses now have no religion, or are of different faiths and spiritual backgrounds, but nurses are duty-bound to respect the differences. The best nurses treat each and every patient as if they are a relative or loved one. And caring for dying patients is the most creative aspect of nursing. The language of spirituality is a way of putting into words something we don't understand. The rituals that we perform may be different from one family to the next, but it is in the act of having respect for these individualities that shared humanity is expressed. Nurses have to honour the spirituality of their patients, however it is expressed, sometimes forcibly suppressing their own beliefs. Nurses have been struck off for praying for patients, for example, with hospitals stating that they have a duty to provide care, without offering unsolicited views of their beliefs. I have worked with nurses who could no longer hide their belief in God than pretend they are flying elephants. It is part of the fabric of who they are, and why they nurse.

Like all nurses, I am taught a working knowledge of all religions: the beliefs associated with illness and disease, suffering and death. But the classroom is no place to learn spiritual care. I learn about Islam not from a nursing textbook, but from my patient who is Muslim, and who asks, before he dies, that his face be turned to the right, towards Mecca. And from his family – a constant stream of people who come and visit – and his obvious delight in seeing them, despite his pain. I learn that his family trust God's will more than they trust the words of the doctors, and how withdrawal-of-care conversations are the most difficult of all, regardless of religion.

My lessons about Jehovah's Witnesses are particularly hard. A young mother is bleeding to death in A&E. She refuses the blood that will save her, and we must let her die for her beliefs. The level of respect that a nurse must have for a patient's own spiritual beliefs can, in some cases, mean that a patient will die. Caring for the person is, and should be, increasingly holistic, but occasionally caring for the person's mind means that their body will die.

When my daughter is five months old I return to work on the Paediatric Intensive-Care Unit. Her dad drops her at nursery when it opens at 8 a.m. (I have left home by 6.30) and I collect her at 6 p.m. Being away from her makes me wake every night in a cold guilt-sweat, but being a mother makes me a different nurse. I start to notice the little things that make a big difference. The bereavement nurse on the ward has always been important to me, but suddenly she is vital, and I respect her in a way that is difficult to articulate. She has children, too, and spends her days helping families who are losing theirs, or have lost them. She helps the staff, from the junior nurses like Savi, who spill emotion into the room, to the consultants who have closed themselves to it. She is an expert interpreter: 'What the doctor is saying is that we can't do any more for Sarah. But what he means is that we can't save your child's body. He has tried his very best. We all have. There is more we can do, still. For Sarah and for you. I am here, and I will be with you, and we will make memories over these next few days. We will make sure that Sarah is not in pain any more, and is comforted and peaceful; and you will get to hold her and be there for her before she dies and afterwards. And I will be right there with you. I am with you.'

The mortuary is where we all end up, but is a place that is unimaginable to most people. I held my breath on my first visit there, and went through one set of doors to another set of doors, to stand in front of stacks of white fridges. The white strip lights and the white fridges and the white walls made everything seem stark and unreal. Too clinical. The opposite of nature. There was no smell at all – none of what normally surrounds the hospital: bleach, sweat, blood, jasmine, urine, aftershave, lavender hand-cream, mint sweets, cigarette smoke in unwashed hair, alcohol gel, shit.

The mortuary smells of nothing. It is the least spooky place you can imagine. If ghosts exist, they don't stay in mortuaries. There is literally no life there. Nothingness. 'One minute we are here,' a mortuary technician shrugs on my first visit, 'then we are gone.'

The process, when a patient gets to the mortuary, varies between hospitals, but goes something like this: the porters are supposed to hoist the body onto a trolley, if sliding isn't possible, then label and document it, and then close the fridge. For bariatric (obese) patients – who are becoming more and more frequent – there are special fridges, walk-ins, where no lifting or handling is required. For babies, another smaller fridge area, and it's usually the nurses, or midwives, who carry them down. If the foetus dies at less than twenty-four weeks, then the body is not registered as dead. 'How can we grieve – we don't even have a death certificate?'

I am no longer squeamish about these things. I am used to life and death, and everything in between. But the coldness of skin on a body pulled from a mortuary fridge is difficult to describe, and forget. Death – like life – has phases, and often by the time a body gets pulled from a mortuary fridge, for a family visit or for a burial or cremation, or (as is frequent in hospitals) for a post-mortem, the body little resembles the person who lived in it. Faces change; skin changes colour. A person's body becomes smaller and waxier.

The mortuary, though, is also where I've witnessed fearless love close up. I've had a horrible week worrying about my lack of money as an NHS nurse: impending bills that I have no means to pay, a car that doesn't start. I have small children who are full of cold and sore throats, and I've sent them to nursery and school respectively, dosed up with Calpol and Nurofen, and am expecting concerned phone calls requesting that I collect them – an impossibility as a nurse in charge on a busy shift.

Halfway through my shift, I escort a mother to see her dead son. I remember her shaking beside me as we walk into the room where Zachary lies wrapped in a soft blanket, in a casket on a trolley. I remember thinking how selfish and small my own worries are. The room is very cramped and is next door to the mortuary. She leans over her son and whispers something that I cannot hear. It is a private moment, and I stand as far back as the room will allow. But then she walks back a few steps and pulls me next to her, clutching my hand. She doesn't cry. She simply looks at him and traces the shape of his face with her thumb. Zachary looks smaller, and his warm, dark skin has turned dull. I know him well. I've nursed him for months, and have spent the last few days preparing for his death. Along with the children's bereavement nurse, we spent the time he was dying cutting a lock of his hair, painting his foot golden. I took a footprint, photographed him with his mum, and played his favourite music around the clock.

'You look peaceful now, my son. No more pain. No more surgery. No more hospitals.' She notices that I am crying and shaking. She pulls the blanket away from him and runs her hand over his body, his tummy, knees, feet. 'You got kids? I never asked you.'

I nod, trying not to sob. My ice-heart crashes.

She looks down for the longest time, touches the bottom of his foot, the gold paint still there. 'Then we are both blessed.'

13

And the Flesh of the
Child Grew Warm

*Don't ever underestimate the capacity of a human being who
is determined to do something.*

Edna Adan Ismail

It's my last day as a nurse and I walk back over the bridge
towards the hospital, watching the water change from green
to blue to grey. I hold on to the colours. I am forty years old,
no longer the skinny girl with a shell against her ear. But
nursing has helped me to listen hard, and finally I can hear
nothing and everything at the same time. My shadow has
jagged edges, and still it dances.

I want to stretch out time, make every last moment of
my final shift count. But as soon as I get to the office the
crash bleep goes off straightaway. I run to find a man has
died unexpectedly in patient transport. There is a nurse I
don't recognise sitting on him, her legs astride his large body;
she is pressing down on his chest, as hard as she can – his
ribs will break. A large pool of sweat V-necks her scrub top,
crescent-moons her armpits. My colleague, Xuan, kneels by
the patient's side, flicks her swinging security ID behind her

back and opens the portable defibrillator, the red shock-box starts talking as soon as she lifts the lid:

'Attach the pads to the patient's chest.

'Plug in the pads next to the flashing light.

'Analysing.

'Shock required.

'Stand clear.'

Xuan talks over the machine, loudly. She knows that people do not listen to machines. 'Come off the chest – it's analysing. Okay, stand clear: we need to shock. Oxygen away, people away.' All the time she is talking, Xuan looks at the patient and sweeps her hand, using her body as well as her voice to keep her colleagues safe from the electricity. Recently, in a London teaching hospital, a nurse accidentally shocked another nurse. There is a theoretical risk that if someone is touching the patient, or even a bag of fluid attached to them, when the shock is delivered, they could end up in cardiac arrest.

Trust in strangers is everything during medical emergencies, for patients and staff alike. The history of the word 'trust' has much in common with the principles of nursing. It came, in Middle English, from 'protection', from the Old Norse word for 'help' and from the Dutch for 'comfort'. Patients must trust their nurses; nurses must trust the doctors, and each other. But nurses must also trust their own ability and limitations. Nurses must know themselves.

After my years of experience, I trust my judgement most of the time. I trust that I've seen it – whatever 'it' is – before, and have reflected on the meaning. I am able to disregard the rule book (as Benner says, the expert nurse 'no longer relies on principles, rules, or guidelines to connect situations and determine actions') and I am in a position to trust my gut reaction above all things. I trust myself – that voice. But this job requires more than that. I need to place that same level of trust in complete strangers.

Many of the cardiac-arrest teams have never met, before they gather at an emergency event. The recommendation by the Resuscitation Council is that the emergency teams in hospital meet before a shift to discuss roles, in order that levels of experience can be ascertained and tasks distributed appropriately. There are a number of roles during a cardiac arrest: team leaders who should stand at the end of the bed and oversee their staff; chest compressions, defibrillation, scribe, drugs. But in a large and frequently changing hospital, where people have full-time jobs in addition to carrying the cardiac-arrest bleep, meeting beforehand is not possible. Trust is everything, but instinct and experience allow quick judgements to be made about the level of expertise of colleagues. A young doctor with his hands in his pockets is not arrogant, but terrified. A consultant holding the patient's wrist to feel for a pulse – instead of a central pulse from a major artery – and shouting orders is not to be trusted at all, and usually realises very quickly that she is out of her depth and removes herself. An anaesthetist, although busy at the head end with the airway, is trustworthy and almost always brilliant. And the calm doctor (or sometimes nurse) who is not shouting, and who is standing at the end of the bed looking at the whole scene – the one who, despite the urgency of the situation, has introduced themselves and said hello, and has asked the names of the team – is to be trusted the most. The most brilliant and experienced doctors I've ever worked with are certainly the calmest, and seem to become even calmer in difficult life-or-death situations.

I watch a consultant let a junior doctor botch many a task, without taking over, knowing that their level of skill will fix any issues, but also that the doctor will not learn without the botches. I'd trust that consultant with my life – with the life of my children. We let things get dangerously close to the edge, as nurses and doctors, while allowing junior members of staff to take too long accessing veins or getting a good seal on a bag valve mask, the patient's chest unmoving, no oxygen getting into their lungs and therefore their brain, as we calmly readjust the hands of the junior nurse or doctor around a patient's face. It is trust in ourselves that enables us to walk right to the cliff edge and know at which point we need to step in, before somebody dies or at least dies more quickly than they would otherwise have done.

The patient-transport area is full, although a porter has found a screen and put it haphazardly around the team who are assembling around the patient. A nurse has appeared from another department and is wheeling out those who are waiting in wheelchairs in patient transport. 'You don't need to see this,' she says.

Xuan is counting thirty compressions, two breaths. No doubt singing in her head to keep time, as we teach it: 'Lady Gaga'. 'Nelly the Elephant' is now considered too slow.

One of the patients in the waiting area is filming on a phone, another is shouting that he has been waiting for a taxi for forty minutes. People seem numb to such catastrophic events in front of them. This is new, something I've only noticed in the last five years or so.

When the crash call goes off in Xuan's pocket, she carries on: she's taken over the chest compressions and is now the one sweating. 'Split the team,' she says, knowing that the call could be a faint in the phlebotomy department or a heart attack in Majors, a relative having an anaphylactic – severe allergic – reaction to peanuts. It could be a call to any one of the five cardiac-arrest teams I work on: trauma, neonatal, obstetric, paediatric or adult. I take out my bleep and run. It turns out to be a senior doctor who has collapsed in the lift. There are enough people on hand to stabilise him and get him to a cardiac ward. Much later on, I hear that he survived; the man in patient transport survived, too.

'You look surprised,' Xuan says.

'Not questioning your excellent chest compressions, merely that it's unusual.'

The survival rate for cardiac arrests in UK hospitals is less than 20 per cent; with a slow decline and co-morbidities (other medical conditions), illnesses and diseases, of course the likelihood of survival – particularly intact – of a cardiac arrest in hospital is abysmal. And, despite our advances in technology and training, we can't seem to improve much on the numbers. It appears that when your time is up, it's up, regardless. Children have even less chance. If they have an asystolic – flatline – cardiac arrest and suffer from a 'flat trace' (a common cardiac-arrest rhythm, of the four rhythms possible in children), then they have just a 5 per cent survival rate. But of those 5 per cent, only 1 per cent will be neurologically intact – that is, they will not suffer irreparable brain damage.

However, in a Las Vegas casino, people have a 75 per cent cardiac-arrest survival rate. This is hypothesised in a number of ways: people are generally well (you'd not agree, if you'd visited a Las Vegas casino and seen people suffering chest pains, but going on holiday anyway); the security staff are trained in how to do chest compressions, and their job depends on them passing regular assessments every four months; people are being continuously watched in case of cheating, so the collapse is witnessed and chest compressions – and, if necessary, shocks – are administered immediately; and, according to many of my colleagues, oxygen is piped into the casino's atmosphere to keep everyone awake.

Most resuscitation experts attest that it is the quality of the chest compressions that makes the most impact on whether someone survives a cardiac arrest. The reason security guards in Las Vegas are given training every four months is because research suggests that we forget clinical skills after this time. In hospitals, the nursing staff are given basic life-support training every year, sometimes every two years and, in some trusts, three-yearly, despite the guidance and recommendations from the Resuscitation Council. It saves money, too, not to offer cardiac-arrest training to children in our schools, although in Scandinavia where this is practised, the out-of-hospital cardiac-arrest survival rate is 30 per cent, whereas ours is more like 10 per cent. Maybe more regular training would improve the figures. More funding. The cost of saving a life.

The man in patient transport is lucky. Xuan is telling me the details at the end of the shift, as she gets changed behind a makeshift screen in our ramshackle office. I get a flash of her tattoo as she pokes her head around the side. The crash bleep goes off again.

'I'll go, so you can handover,' I say. I run out onto the link corridor, past the bereavement office and down the stairs, two at a time. I am out of breath as I pass the children's outpatients area, where a small boy wearing thick glasses has his face pressed up against the glass. I run past Ophthalmology, and the smell of air freshener; past the cardiac clinic, where I can see the machines lined up against the wall; and a man wearing jeans and a thick jumper slopes past, looking just like my dad.

I see him everywhere. For a long time I go through the motions of life. I am in the operating theatre – somewhere between worlds. But time flies; Gladys was right. Days become weeks and months and years, and the children and I survive an awful time. Nursing, and my children, provide me with such kindness. Occasionally the blood from the umbilical cord flows both ways. Time always changes night to day, eventually.

I take large breaths as I run past the psychiatric offices, and the ward for long-term patients requiring breathing machines; and the ever-expanding private-patients' wing and the dementia ward; the stroke unit, the plastic-surgery ward, the burns centre, the heart centre, neurosurgical intensive care, the sexual-health wing, the breast-cancer clinic. I run past the blood-testing rooms and the dental theatres. The mortuary is underneath me, and the labour wards are above. And everything blurs. And I hear a baby crying.

The crash bleep pulls me to the car park outside Accident and Emergency, where the ambulances are beginning to queue in a line and the paramedics are working on patients who are seriously injured or dying, and too ill to be transported into the hospital.

There's an invisible line around each hospital within which the internal crash team can respond; outside this, an ambulance must be called. The hospital car park lies within this space, although the patient who had a full-blown cardiac arrest on a bus outside the hospital was beyond the line. It didn't stop my colleague from climbing on him and trying to resuscitate him, though. 'What should I do? Wait eight minutes, or twenty, for an ambulance, and ensure this man is brain-dead?' It doesn't stop the nurses and doctors running towards a terrorist.

I arrive in the car park to find a black cab, with the driver standing outside it, his face a twist of copper-grey, pointing to the open door. A woman with legs as thick as tree trunks is pushing out a baby. My colleague, an A&E nurse called Beatte, has her hands stretched out, no gloves on, and is about to catch the baby that is already sliding out. 'Quick, help!'

'I don't want no trouble.' The taxi driver is behind me. His meter continues to run. There is blood and shit everywhere.

The woman has her eyes closed and is moaning a kind of non-human moan that I recognise. Groaning. There is a noise like a car going over a large pothole, clunking.

'What's your name?' I ask. But she is far away. I turn to Beatte.

'This is Priscilla,' she says. 'The porters are bringing blankets, but we need them yesterday.' Her voice is breaking. She is not a midwife. And nor am I. This is so far beyond our experience. Anything can happen.

I look at the taxi driver. 'Give me your coat.'

He pulls it off and I put the coat underneath my colleague's hands, which are by now covered in all kinds of shit. The baby falls out, quiet. Priscilla screams. A crowd gathers. I look up for a second. All of life is here, in this car park, in this hospital. People from all corners of the world: vulnerable, frail and human. We are living history.

A young, bald man has pushed his drip-stand over to the scene. He wears pyjamas and has a central line hanging from his chest, which is so thin that his ribs look like a xylophone. Cancer. 'Do you need help?' he asks.

'It's a baby,' the taxi driver is shouting. 'A baby.'

And the baby screams a beautiful scream, changing from a dead thing to living in a matter of a breath. The blankets arrive. I check the baby, its colour, tone and posture, listen to its running, strong heart with the small side of my stethoscope. A perfectly fast beat. Running towards life. I give her back to the mother. 'Congratulations, you have a daughter.'

She sits slightly upright, her legs an open, bloody mess, the cord still connecting mother and baby, her body shaking. She laughs and looks at the baby, then up at the taxi driver. 'God is great.'

We find a wheelchair, and help Priscilla and the new baby out of the taxi into the chair, and cover them with blankets. Never before has a woman smiled so broadly. I stand beside them and walk as Beatte pushes the chair. The baby looks at her mum with eyes bigger than the sky.

The crash bleep goes off again as we walk: 'Trauma Call, Accident and Emergency.'

'I'll run ahead.' I smile at Priscilla, but she's too busy looking at her new daughter to notice me. Which is exactly as it should be.

I run. My heart runs faster, too. A&E is frightening. It reminds us that life is fragile. And what could be more frightening than that? A&E teaches us that we are small: despite our best efforts, we can't predict who will lose their husband; who will have a heart attack or a stroke; who will deliver a baby with a complex heart condition; who will lose a newborn to infection or deliver prematurely. We don't know which one of us will develop a lifelong mental illness. We don't know who among us will abuse their children. We can't predict which of us will need our bed changing because we are incontinent, and who will change that bed. We don't know who will suffer diabetes, asthma, sepsis; who will be burnt in a fire. We don't know who will get cancer, or where the wind will blow.

Even now I'm afraid when I push open the door to Accident and Emergency. So let us go in together. I take a deep breath. If you come with me, then anything is bearable. Take my hand. Hold my hand tightly. Let us fling open the door and find whatever we find, face all the horror and beauty of life. Let us really live. Together, our hands will not shake.

Afterword

Life has been an unexpected whirlwind since publication of *The Language of Kindness*. I've been fortunate enough to travel across the country and even the world, appearing in newspapers, magazines, on radio and TV. My children have almost forgotten what I look like in real life – and would much rather I was home making them cheesy beans on toast. But they do love to hear about the people I've met along the way.

There has been no greater joy for me than meeting readers and hearing other people's ordinary and extraordinary stories. Speaking to the nurses and doctors and patients who have read my book and found some commonality between our lives and experiences has been a true honour. People have reached out to me in person, by letter, email and on social media and what has been astonishing, reassuring and life-affirming is that everyone's lives hold so many similarities; we are all such a mixture of tragedy and joy. It thrills me to hear from readers and it is humbling to know that my words have meant something to people, have touched them and reminded them – and me – that we are all connected.

A woman with only weeks to live sought me out after an event, and thanked me for raising not just the profile of nurses, but also the importance of kindness. I visited her at home and we talked for hours about the things that are most important, in the end. The things that will matter to all of us. The precious nature of this life, of nature, and most of all, of love. A nurse who was 101 years old came to a book event from her care home to say thank you. *It's hard to get the job of a nurse into words,* she told me. *Well done.* This one nod of approval from a lifelong nurse meant more than I can say. I've met thousands of nurses and I hope to meet many more. When I was asked to give the keynote speech at the Royal College of Nursing congress to 3,000 nurses I was suitably terrified. They were a tough crowd: experienced nurses who had a tendency to slow clap politicians. The entire front row was asleep when I started. But afterwards I received a standing ovation. Looking up at the end of my speech, with my heart still pounding in my ears, to see my nursing family on their feet – it meant everything.

At that event, as at all the others, I was asked difficult questions. Student nurses and medical students wanted advice about training or career. Members of the public and patients, and sometimes politicians, asked me about what we can do to help the nursing crisis, the NHS, society. I don't consider myself qualified to answer these big questions – or rather, I've always felt there are far more qualified people. But with the platform that the book has enabled me to have, I feel duty-bound to highlight the significance of nursing and what we risk losing if we don't have enough nurses. I want to share my thoughts about nursing recruitment and the scrapping of the nursing bursary when we are 42,000 nurses short in the UK. Retention is the real issue. With no bursary, a newly qualified nurse starting out with £60,000 worth of debt is much less likely to manage a career-long commitment to nursing. And we're seeing this across the board; nurses are leaving the NHS faster than they're joining. NHS staff are the biggest users of payday loans, and nurses in full-time employment are accessing charity hardship funds simply to buy food, to pay for heating, to survive. Paying our nurses properly while they train and beyond is my most pressing concern. Perhaps my time as a nurse when I found my ten-year-old daughter trying to sellotape a large hole in her school shoes, because she knew I did not have any money to buy her new ones, qualifies me to give that advice.

People ask me about mental health, my own and others'. We don't pay much attention to the mental health of nurses. I remember when I first started out as a nurse I tried to make my stomach hard, to deny my feelings, to remain detached. I thought I was somehow safeguarding the professional relationship between nurse and patient. Nursing is the best friend of empathy. Kindness, compassion and sympathy are all essential aspects of being a nurse, but to be a great nurse you need empathy, and that's the part that takes a chunk of your soul. I used to think that feeling empathy without necessarily showing it was the safest way to be, for both nurse and patient. But it harms. Nurses go on a journey with their patients, and it's good for both the patient and the nurse to understand how much that relationship means, and how deeply it is felt. The things that nurses see and touch and smell, the things they hold in their hands and hold in their hearts. Nurses should cry, if they need to cry. Being able to describe the emotional weight that nurses have to carry (and hide) has been very important to me. Talking about the book to readers has been a way of stripping away the barriers between groups of people. I hope it's helped us all celebrate nursing.

People cry at my events. They come up afterwards and cry in front of me until I go across to the other side of the signing table and hold them, then they cry some more. People write me letters or emails or tweets to tell me how my losing my dad reminded them so much of losing their dad, or their mum, or their child. I've learnt so much from the nurses and doctors and student nurses and medical students who come to my events. But my book was not about what I thought it was about. 'I lost my dad too,' said a man who had queued up to speak to me after a talk. 'Your book is about grief, it's about the loss of your father.'

He was right, of course. When I acknowledged this everything I thought shifted. Something clicked into place about my relationship with the book, with my writing, with myself.

I thought about his comment when I was on a panel at a recent event at a Waterstones store in London. A woman queued up at the end. She said she was too shy to raise her hand during the Q&A. She wanted to know what the single biggest lesson I'd learnt in my many years as a nurse was. She said she had been a nurse for fifteen years but was finding it so difficult as staffing levels were worse than ever. Despite this she loved learning, every day, about what it means to be human. We talked about all that nursing can teach a person. I spent twenty years, both nursing and writing, searching for answers to the big questions: love, life, death, loss, grief. And nursing taught me that life is completely random, can turn on a dime, and the worst possible things you can ever imagine happen to the best people. The cruelest of people can have the greatest capacity for love, and change is possible in all of us. Right or wrong and good or evil are meaningless without context. I understand all of these things now.

In writing the book, I felt it was therapeutic to share the story of my own life and loss. And it probably was. But I had built up such sophisticated emotional walls that I couldn't even see them myself. As much as I was aware of emotional burnout and compassion fatigue, I had spent twenty years cultivating that professional detachment from my own feelings, keeping everything at arm's length in order to try and protect myself somehow. I was familiar with emotional numbing as a feature of post-traumatic stress disorder. But I didn't recognise it in myself. I laughed and cried like everyone else. But I was numb. And now I am becoming less so, maybe with distance and time, but more likely by listening to other people generously sharing their own lives with me. I have met or heard from dozens of people a week who want to share their own grief, their own stories, what happened to them or their loved ones, and who they lost. This has been re-triggering, taking its toll. Every story I hear hurts. My emotional nerve endings are more exposed than they have been in years. I feel raw and I am more susceptible to the pain I kept at bay for so long. I'm a wreck, but somehow I feel healthier.

I see my dad everywhere. A flash of greying hair and mischievous eyes, a man walking past with the same quick walk, a coat the same colour as his. Another man digging up potatoes in an allotment had me stop in my tracks. I dream of my dad, and when I wake I try desperately to get back to the same dream. I have a jumper of his screwed up in the bottom of my wardrobe that still, even after seven years, smells faintly of him: oranges and bonfires and wet mud and toffee. But it's becoming fainter. I am so anxious that his smell will be gone forever. Nursing taught me so many lessons, but it was grief that taught me something that is the most beautifully, and painfully, true: people don't really ever leave us. Not if we love them enough.

Christie Watson, January 2019

Acknowledgements

With thanks to the champions of kindness:

Sophie Lambert, Juliet Brooke and Clara Farmer.

Anna Stein, Emma Finn, Alexandra McNicoll, Alexander Cochran, Jake Smith-Bosanquet and the team at C+W Agency; Charlotte Humphery, Suzanne Dean, Chloe Healy, Fran Owen, Mari Yamazaki, Sophie Mitchell and the Chatto and Vintage teams; Tim Duggan, Will Wolfslau and the Tim Duggan Books team; Amy Black, Kristin Cochrane and Doubleday Canada; Lucas Telles and Intrinseca; Elise Noerholm, Jeanette Holm and Lindhardt of Ringhof; Fleur d'Harcourt and Flammarion; Zhaoming Zhong, Yume Horikawa and Shanghai Insight Media; Georg Reuchlein, Katharina Fokken and Goldmann; Emanuele Basile and Mondadori; Heleen Buth, Jacqueline de Jong, Lisanne Mathijssen and HarperCollins Holland; Alexandra Matyi and Alexandra Kiado; Gunn Reinertsen, Synnøve Tresselt and Aschehoug; Katarzyna Rudzka, Alicja Galandzij and Marginsey; Sara Wunderly Gomes, Amaia Iglesias and Penguin Random House, Portugal; Rosa Pérez and Plaza & Janes; Pema Maymo Veny and Montse Armengol Díaz and Columna and Grup62; Elin Sennero, Sara Nyström, Johanna Haegerström and Albert Bonniers; Tina Pan and

Locus; Ekaterina Novak and Family Leisure Club Ukraine; Hayakawa Publishing, Nike Books, Azbooka-Atticus, LEDA, Luke Speed, Rebecca Keane, Damien Timmer, Rachel Bennette, Suzanne O'Sullivan, Nathan Filer, Lewis Buxton, Nicola Fisher, Edmund Glynn, Simon and Anne Nadel, Russell Schechter, Jonathan Gibbs and St Mary's University, Sarah Chaney, Janet Davies and the Royal College of Nursing.

Thank you to Cheryl, my dad's nurse, and to all the nurses and doctors I've worked with who have taught me so much about life, death, and everything in between. You are my heroes.

Finally I'd like to thank all the patients I've known over the years. What an extraordinary privilege it was to be your nurse.

Every day, thousands of people rely on the care of nurses, midwives and healthcare assistants. The RCN Foundation gives vital support back to these caring professionals. They safeguard nurses facing hardship by providing advice and support to get their lives back on track. They invest in the future of nursing by funding learning and development opportunities. And they fund innovative nursing-led projects that contribute to improving the health and well-being of the public.

To donate to the RCN Foundation and help to support and strengthen nursing, visit their website:

www.rcnfoundation.org.uk/support_us